Root Eye Dictionary

A "Layman's Explanation" of the eye
and common eye problems

Written and Illustrated by

Timothy Root, M.D.

www.RootEyeDictionary.com

Contents:

Introduction

The Dictionary, A-Z

Extra Stuff

- Abbreviations

- Other Books by Dr. Root

~>Intro~<

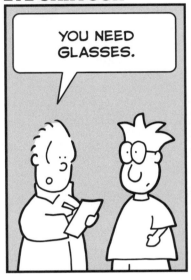

YOU NEED GLASSES.

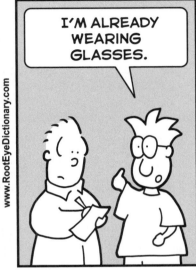

I'M ALREADY WEARING GLASSES.

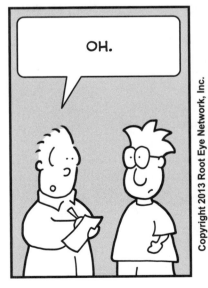

OH.

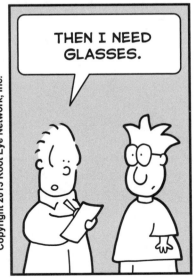

THEN I NEED GLASSES.

www.RootEyeDictionary.com

INTRODUCTION

Greetings and welcome to the Root Eye Dictionary. Inside these pages you will find an alphabetical listing of common eye diseases and visual problems I treat on a day-to-day basis.

Ophthalmology is a field riddled with confusing concepts and nomenclature, so I figured a layman's dictionary might help you "decode" the medical jargon. Hopefully, this explanatory approach helps remove some of the mystery behind eye disease.

With this book, you should be able to:

> 1. Look up any eye "diagnosis" you or your family has been given
>
> 2. Know why you are getting eye "tests"
>
> 3. Look up the ingredients of your eye drops.

As you read any particular topic, you will see that some words are underlined. An underlined word means that I've written another entry for that particular topic. You can flip to that section if you'd like further explanation, though I've attempted to make each entry understandable on its own merit. I'm hoping this approach allows you to learn more about the eye without getting bogged down with minutia ... but if you are interested in a topic, you can dive in as deep as you like!

Even though this book is full of information, I discourage you from trying to diagnose your own eye problems ... or opening your own eye clinic in your garage. Many eye diseases present with similar symptoms and can only be diagnosed by examination under a microscope. When in doubt, it is best to consult with an actual eye doctor. You should look upon this book as supplemental education and NOT as medical advice. With that said, I hope you find this information useful.

Timothy Root, M.D.

Root's Disclaimers

Here are a couple of things to keep in mind as you read this book:

Accuracy: With many of the topics here, I faced a dilemma between factual accuracy and maintaining "understandability." When in doubt, I've decided to err on the side of understandability. You may occasionally find information that is not 100% technically accurate. This is a book designed to improve comprehension through intuitive examples and metaphor. If you need more exact definitions, I can point you toward medical textbooks and journal articles that I've written for this purpose.

Cartoons: A "dictionary" can be a rather boring textbook to read. To keep this book interesting, I've added many cartoons and comic strips. These silly jokes are not meant to downplay eye disease or disrespect patients. Rather, this lighthearted approach is meant to keep this book palatable and easy to read. No offense is intended, and I hope you approach these cartoons with the same good-natured outlook that I had when I illustrated them.

Opinion: If you see another doctor, you may find information in this book that conflicts with what you've been told about the eye. When in doubt, listen to the doctor who has actually examined your eyes. This book reflects my own personal beliefs, medical experiences, and is specific to the greater Daytona Beach area.

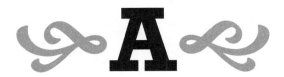

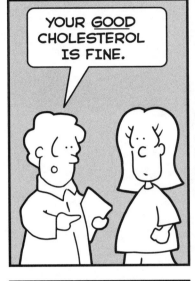

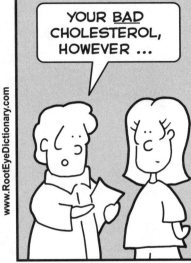

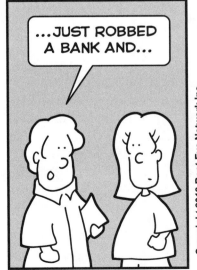

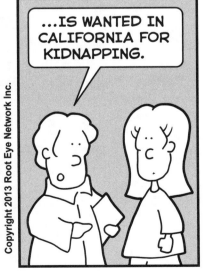

www.RootEyeDictionary.com

Copyright 2013 Root Eye Network Inc.

accommodation. Accommodation is the process by which the eye focuses to see near objects. A normal eye, that is to say, an eye that is neither <u>nearsighted</u> nor <u>farsighted,</u> is naturally focused to see distant objects clearly. To see close-up objects, such as when reading, the flexible <u>lens</u> inside the eye changes shape and becomes "rounder." This process is called accommodation and is quite versatile when young. After the age of 40, however, our lens becomes stiff and accommodation becomes more challenging. We lose our ability to accommodate and we become more dependent on <u>glasses</u> and <u>bifocals</u> with time. This loss of accommodation is called <u>presbyopia</u>.

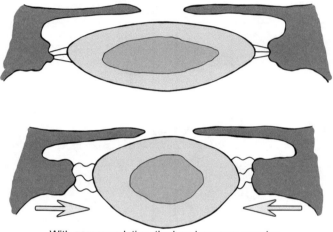

With accommodation, the lens becomes rounder.

acetazolamide. An oral water pill that is used to treat <u>glaucoma</u>. This pill is a diuretic and will dehydrate the body, but it will also dehydrate the eye and decrease eye <u>pressure</u>. This medication is also known as <u>Diamox</u> and is normally used in cases of extremely high eye pressure where we've exhausted our topical eye drop options, or used immediately after other eye surgery to avoid pressure spikes. Don't confuse this with acetomenophine (Tylenol). If you switch these, you might be up all night peeing instead of curing your headache. This pill is also used for people going to high altitudes to avoid mountain sickness. Side effects are minor but can include tingling sensations in the fingers/toes and carbonated soft drinks may taste odd.

Acular. This is an eye drop in the <u>NSAID</u> class of medicines. It is an anti-inflammatory drop with a mechanism similar to Advil or Motrin. It is occasionally used to help with ocular discomfort but mainly used after eye surgery. This class of medicines is good at decreasing the chance of <u>macular edema</u> (retinal swelling) after <u>cataract surgery</u>. It can sting a little going in, however.

acute glaucoma. Acute glaucoma is when the <u>pressure</u> inside the eye goes up suddenly. This usually occurs because of a sudden closure of the drainage "<u>angle</u>" inside the eye. With no drainage, the <u>aqueous</u> humor fluid builds up and causes a spike in eye pressure that can lead to rapid vision loss. Symptoms include extreme eye pain along with nausea and halos seen around lights. Treatment is geared toward lowering the pressure and "breaking the attack," often with a laser, eye drops, and diuretic pills like <u>Diamox</u>. Acute glaucoma is less common in the USA as most people with glaucoma have <u>chronic "open-angle" glaucoma</u>. If an eye appears to be at risk for having an attack, then we will sometimes perform a prophylactic laser procedure called a laser peripheral iridotomy (<u>LPI</u>) to decrease the likelihood of this problem.

acyclovir. An antiviral pill used for viral infections such as <u>shingles</u> (chicken pox) and <u>herpetic eye disease</u>. This medication is cheap and effective, but requires a lot of pills to get the correct dosing. A similar medicine we use is called <u>Valtrex</u> (<u>valacyclovir</u>). Some people with these recurring infections will take a maintenance dose of acyclovir to decrease the chance of a new outbreak.

Adie's pupil. This is a neurologic disorder in which one eye becomes dilated. Most patients have no symptoms or visual complaints, but a friend points out that one of their pupils is now much larger than the other. Also, the <u>pupil</u> does not seem to constrict normally with light. An Adie's pupil usually occurs from damage to one of the nerve clusters behind the eye (inside the eye socket) that controls pupil constriction. This damage can occur from an otherwise harmless viral infection such as a common cold. The problem is usually temporary and goes away after a few months. The opposite condition is called <u>Horner's syndrome</u>. Horner's causes pupil constriction and is potentially dangerous.

after-cataract. This is a cloudy membrane that forms on the back surface of an <u>implant</u> lens inside the eye after <u>cataract surgery</u>. This opacity can form months or years after a successful cataract operation and can cause blur and glare symptoms (similar to the original <u>cataract</u>). These "after cataracts" are not a complication from cataract surgery, but rather a continued proliferation of tissue inside the eye (similar to scar tissue). After-cataracts are easy to treat with a <u>laser</u>. A <u>YAG capsulotomy</u> can be performed to create a hole through the opaque membrane. This is a simple, painless procedure, and once performed the "after cataract" does not typically reoccur.

Alaway. An effective over-the-counter allergy drop. Alaway contains the medicine <u>ketotifen</u> and is usually used twice a day. Allergy drops are good for itching and swelling, and can make the eye feel less sensitive. Alaway and <u>Zaditor</u> (which contains the same active ingredient) are two of my favorite over-the-counter allergy drops.

allergic conjunctivitis. The eyes are particularly sensitive to environmental allergens. Symptoms are usually bilateral, with both eyes being itchy and puffy. <u>Eyelid</u> swelling can be so bad that you look like you've been in a fight ... we call these "allergic shiners." Treatment for allergic <u>conjunctivitis</u> involves cool compresses, antihistamine <u>allergy drops</u>, and occasionally mild <u>steroid</u> drops.

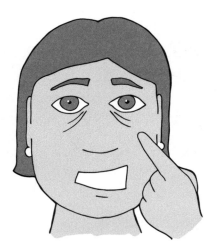

allergy drops. Allergy drops are commonly used to treat ocular itching and swelling. There are several types of allergy drops on the market. The first generation antihistamine drops like <u>Opcon-A</u> are effective but tend to give short-lived relief. Second generation antihistamines like <u>Alaway</u>/<u>Zaditor</u> are more effective and what I recommend for most of my patients. Prescription strength allergy drops are also available such as <u>Bepreve</u>, <u>Pataday</u>, and <u>Lastacaft</u>.

Alphagan. A glaucoma drop used to lower eye pressure. This drop went generic so many people have switched to generic brimonidine or moved up to Alphagan P.

Alphagan P. This is a glaucoma eye drop designed to lower eye pressure. It is actually a "new" formulation of brimonidine that has a lower concentration of active drug and a less harsh preservative in it. Despite the decreased concentration, the drop appears to have the same efficacy as the old Alphagan but with less irritating side effects.

Alrex. A mild steroid eye drop. Useful in cases of ocular inflammation and irritation. This drop has the same ingredient (loteprednol) as Lotemax but with a third of the steroid concentration. By reducing the steroid concentration, this decreases the chance of untoward reactions such as premature cataract formation and glaucoma pressure spikes.

ALT. This stands for Argon Laser Trabeculoplasty and is a laser procedure designed to lower the eye pressure in people with glaucoma. This procedure involves using a "hot" laser to burn spots into the trabecular meshwork (the drainage filter of the eye). By doing this, scar tissue forms that opens up the meshwork and creates better flow. While effective and well tolerated, the pressure improvements of ALT tend to wear off in a couple of years. The procedure can only be done once because of the scar formation. ALT is largely being replaced by a similar procedure called SLT. With SLT a "cold" YAG laser is used to create similar spots on the trabecular meshwork but instead of creating heat-induced scars, the drainage cells are merely stimulated. This promotes better flow through the drain without creating permanent tissue damage. This means that SLT can be repeated if it wears off. SLT is slowly becoming first-line therapy for many doctors treating glaucoma.

amblyopia. Also known as "lazy eye." Amblyopia occurs at a young age from disuse when an eye doesn't see well. A child's visual nervous system is still developing until age seven. If during this developmental period, one eye has poorer vision, the "brain wiring" for that eye does not form as strongly as the better eye. This can occur because of early nearsightedness or early farsightedness or from other visual problems such as congenital cataract. This imbalance can also occur if the eyes are in poor alignment (like being cross-eyed). If detected early, amblyopia can be reversed. This is typically accomplished with glasses and patching therapy - by patching the "good eye" closed, this forces the lazy eye to "work" and reform its wiring. There is no way to fix a lazy eye in adulthood as the brain wiring has already formed and the amblyopic eye will never see quite as well.

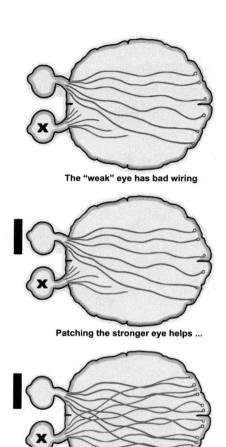

The "weak" eye has bad wiring

Patching the stronger eye helps ...

... allowing weak connections to grow.

amiodarone. This is a commonly used oral medication that is used to help with abnormal rhythms of the heart (arrhythmias). While effective, amiodarone can occasionally cause changes in the eye. One of these changes is "corneal verticillata," which are pigment deposits in the clear cornea that can be seen with the slit lamp microscope. These corneal changes rarely cause any appreciable vision problems, but if severe may prompt a change in medication.

amphotericin B. An antifungal medicine that can be compounded (see fortified antibiotics) and used to treat fungal eye infections. There are not many antifungal eye medications out there - the only other eye drop easily available is Natamycin.

Amsler grid. A checkered pattern used at home for detecting retinal distortions, such as from macular degeneration or an epiretinal membrane. To use, a patient is instructed to look at the central dot while covering an eye. If the surrounding lines are missing or look distorted, then the surface of the retina (which acts like "film in a camera") may be distorted as well. This prompts further evaluation and retinal scans like an OCT to find these problems. My patients are often sent home with a copy of this grid to monitor their vision at home. Stop by my office for a free copy if you don't already have one.

anesthetic drops. There are several drops we use to anesthetize the surface of the eye. The most common one is called proparacaine, though we occasionally use tetracaine. These drops are very similar to the "novacaine" that a dentist uses ... but fortunately we don't have to use a needle to apply it! Numbing drops make it easier to check eyes pressure using applanation tonometry. We also use these drops prior to cataract surgery to minimize discomfort. Unfortunately, anesthetic eye drops are not safe for home use. The medications are toxic to the corneal surface when used repeatedly and will keep surface wounds from healing. For pain, we prescribe ointments, bandage contact lenses, and can even patch an eye shut if needed (see patching).

angle. In regards to the eye, the "angle" usually refers to the drainage angle inside the eye where excess ocular fluid (aqueous) is reabsorbed back into the blood stream. This angle is located at the intersection of the iris and the white sclera of the eye ... in other words, in a 360-degree ring where the "white" of the eye meets the "colored part" of the eye. If this angle closes down, then you can have an angle-closure glaucoma, also known as acute glaucoma.

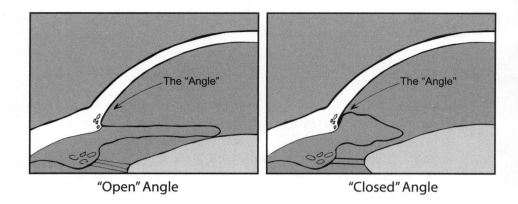

"Open" Angle   "Closed" Angle

anisocoria. This is when the pupils are of unequal size. Many people have slightly different sized pupils and this is considered normal. Large differences between the eye is not normal, however. See <u>dilated pupil</u> for more information.

anterior chamber. This is the fluid-filled space in the front part of the eye, located immediately behind the cornea but in front of the iris. This "chamber" is filled with clear <u>aqueous</u> fluid and easy to examine by the doctor using the <u>slit lamp microscope</u> in the office. In cases of trauma or <u>iritis</u>, the anterior chamber may be filled with inflammatory cells that can be detected in the office. In more severe cases of trauma, blood can fill this space ... this is called a <u>hyphema</u>. If you have <u>acute glaucoma</u>, the anterior chamber can be shallow as the <u>aqueous</u> fluid cannot drain out properly.

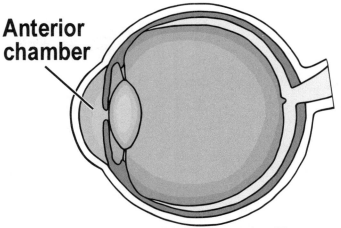

Anterior chamber

The "anterior chamber" is the fluid-filled front portion of the eye.
This fluid is called "aqueous."

antibiotic. This usually refers to a drop or pill that is designed to kill or decrease the proliferation of bacteria. The eye is well protected from infection by the conjunctiva and the corneal epithelium. In addition, the tear film contains antimicrobials and the tear flow itself tends to wash away pathogens. The eye also harbors a host of non-pathogenic bacteria that competitively prohibit new bacteria growth. However, these eye defenses can be breached by trauma, improper tearing, or contact lens wear and lead to an infection. Topical antibiotics work best for the eye given the avascular nature of the cornea.

anti-VEGF. This is a class of medicines that are designed to combat neovascularization inside the eye and decrease blood vessel leakage. They are usually used for treating problems like macular edema, caused by wet macular degeneration, though occasionally they are used for treating swelling from other sources such as diabetic retinopathy or central retinal vein occlusion. These medicines work by decreasing leakage of fluid across abnormal blood vessels in the retina. The original anti-VEGF medication used was the injection medicine Avastin which was originally formulated for combating colon cancer. Lucentis and Eylea are newer anti-VEGF medications that may be more effective with less systemic side effects, but are quite costly when compared to Avastin. Refer to the entries on VEGF and neovascularization to better understand how these medications work.

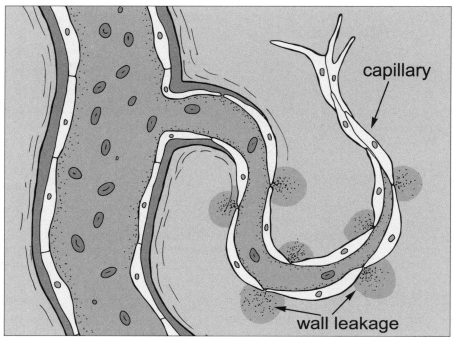
Anti-VEGF medications target leaky capillaries in the retina.

aphakia. This is when the natural lens has been removed from the eye (such as after <u>cataract surgery</u>) but has not been replaced with a new lens <u>implant</u>. In the early days of eye surgery, cataracts were removed but not replaced with anything. The vision was better but "aphakic people" required thick coke-bottle glasses to see well. Today, most people receive a new implant so aphakia is rare. Most people with aphakic eyes have had some kind of trauma or complicated cataract surgery that precludes the placement of a modern lens implant.

applanation tonometry. This is a method for checking the <u>pressure</u> inside the eye. The eyeball is a closed ball of fluid so that there is no good way to measure the internal pressure of the eyeball directly. However, we can estimate the eye pressure by pushing on the surface of the eye and feeling "how hard" is seems. This is similar to kicking a car tire to estimate the air pressure inside. With applanation tonometry, a flat probe is pushed onto the surface of the cornea (the clear window that makes up the front of the eye). The probe is pushed hard enough to flatten a small round area of the <u>cornea</u>. By looking at the size of the circle flattened, and examining the amount of pressure used, the internal eye pressure can be calculated. The machine we use for this is called a Goldmann Applanation Tonometer. It is attached to the <u>slit lamp microscope</u> and it looks like a blue light when in use. You don't feel this measurement as we use <u>anesthetic drops</u> ahead of time.

aqueous

. The aqueous "humor" is the fluid that fills the front part of the eye (the <u>anterior chamber</u>). This clear fluid maintains the shape of the eye and affects the eye <u>pressure</u>. <u>Glaucoma</u> can occur if the pressure gets too high, and most glaucoma treatments are geared toward regulating the production and drainage of the aqueous fluid. Several structures in the eye, such as the <u>cornea</u> and <u>lens</u>, contain no blood vessels and rely on the aqueous humor to provide them with nutritional support.

arcus senilis

. This is a white haze or ring on the cornea that occurs with age. The <u>cornea</u> is the clear window that makes up the front of the eye. This living tissue has no blood vessels running through it because it needs to be perfectly clear. To get its nutrition, the cornea depends upon the <u>tear film</u> on the outside, the <u>aqueous</u> fluid on the inside, and blood vessels on the <u>sclera</u> (the white of the eye) that run right up to the edge of cornea before stopping. Lipid and cholesterol fats travel in our blood stream, and over a lifetime, can leach out of the blood vessels and deposit themselves in a ring in the cornea. This white ring is called arcus senilis and is a normal aging change that has no effect on vision. When I see this in only one eye (or in a young person) I start looking into other problems such as circulation or cholesterol abnormalities.

AREDS Study

. This stands for the Age-Related Eye Disease Study. This large study was conducted to study the effects of vitamin supplements in slowing the progression of <u>macular degeneration</u>. The study showed that certain antioxidants were more helpful, such as Vitamin A, Vitamin C, and Vitamin E and the metals zinc and copper (cupric acid). While these vitamins are found in a healthy diet, the high doses used in the AREDS trial were much higher than normal multivitamin tablets and are difficult to obtain through normal food intake. Therefore, additional oral pill supplements are recommended in anyone with signs of macular degeneration. While vitamins are generally safe, there are a few caveats you should keep in mind. If you are a smoker, you should NOT take any supplements with Vitamin A (beta-carotene) as this has been associated with higher rates of lung cancer. You really shouldn't be smoking, as smoking has been found to speed macular degeneration in its own right. Also, there is some controversy over whether dietary zinc might slightly increase the risk of prostate cancer for men, but most authorities seem to think it safe. Both of these problems are being studied in the AREDS 2 Study.

AREDS 2 Study. This is the latest study searching for additional supplements that slow down macular degeneration progression. In the original AREDS Study, researchers found that Vitamin A (beta-carotene), C, E and the metals zinc and copper were helpful in slowing the progression of vision loss. However, there are many more supplements out there that have been theorized to be healthy for the eye. The AREDS2 clinical trial finished in 2012 and the results are only now coming to light. It appears that the omega-3 fatty acids (DHA and EPA) had little effect on the eye, despite their known cardiac and stroke benefits. However, the plant pigments lutein and zeaxanthin were found to be helpful and may be a good replacement for beta-carotene (which is contraindicated in smokers because of increased lung cancer risk). AREDS 2 vitamins are beginning to show up on the shelves and are safe for most people. Vitamin packaging can be confusing. If you are a smoker or have had lung cancer, be sure to read the contents and avoid any vitamins with beta-carotene.

ARMD. This stands for Age-Related Macular Degeneration and is just another way of saying macular degeneration. See the entry on macular degeneration for more details.

artificial tears. These are rewetting drops that can be bought over the counter and used for dry eye. Artificial tears are produced by many manufacturers and are essentially all the same. The only real difference between them is what preservative is used to keep the drops sterile. This preservative is crucial for keeping the drops fresh and free of environmental bacteria. However, the preservative itself (especially BAK)

can be irritating to the eye if the drops are used too often. Preservative-free artificial tears are available that eliminate this problem. They come in single-use disposable plastic dispensers and can be used as often as needed.

A-scan. This is a type of ultrasound used on the eye and is primarily used to measure the length of the eyeball. This measurement is needed prior to cataract surgery so that we can calculate the correct implant power for the replacement lens. A-scan ultrasound can be very precise but only focuses on one parameter - the length of the eye. This is in contrast to B-scan ultrasound, which actually produces an image of the interior structures of the eye (and is more akin to the fetal ultrasound used in pregnancy).

asteroid hyalosis. This is a harmless condition where calcium soap deposits form inside the vitreous fluid that fills the back of the eye. During an eye exam, these little specks glow brightly under the microscope - in fact, the inside of the eye looks like a blizzard or snow globe. Despite the impressive microscopic appearance, these deposits cause little visual symptoms though some people complain of more floaters than normal. Asteroid hyalosis is primarily an incidental finding seen during an eye exam and not an indicator of any problems. If there are enough floaters to obstruct vision, a vitrectomy surgery could be considered, but this is rarely indicated. Asteroid hyalosis is mainly of interest to eye doctors. We may grab a medical student or two to show you off, though!

asthenopia. This is a fancy word for eye strain or discomfort. There are many causes for eye strain, including incorrect glasses, motility problems (the eyes out of alignment), or even from surface irritation such as dry eye.

astigmatism. This is when the eye is oval in shape. Normally the surface of the cornea is perfectly round like a basketball. Some people's cornea is shaped more like a football ... that is to say, the cornea is steep along one axis and shallow along the other. This is called astigmatism and

is completely normal. It is easy to fix astigmatism using <u>glasses</u>, as the "mirror image" of your eye's football can be ground into your glasses and aligned to give good vision. There are also <u>toric contacts</u> that can fix astigmatism though they are a little harder to fit as contacts spin on the surface of the eye. Finally, there are now <u>toric implants</u> used in <u>cataract surgery</u>. These implants have the football shape ground in ahead of time. During surgery, we rotate this implant inside the eye until it perfectly balances out and eliminates your eye's natural astigmatism.

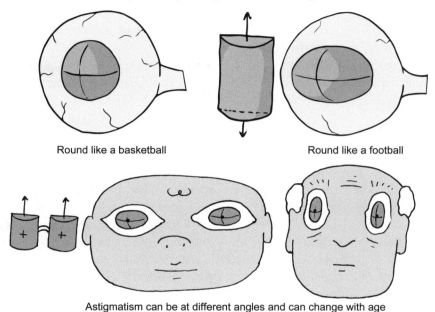

Round like a basketball   Round like a football

Astigmatism can be at different angles and can change with age

atropine. A powerful dilating drop. This drop is so powerful, in fact, that your eye may be dilated for a week after its use. This is also a <u>cycloplegia</u> drop typically given in cases of ocular inflammation (<u>iritis</u>) to help with pain control by temporarily paralyzing the <u>iris</u> muscle inside the eye. The drop is often used after retina surgery for similar reasons, but also because atropine appears to have some anti-inflammatory properties in its own right. Young children can take a long time to dilate, so this drop is occasionally used at home to dilate a child prior to their eye exam. The blurring effect can also be used as a kind of "chemical <u>patching</u>" in cases of <u>amblyopia</u> (lazy eye) - especially useful in a child who won't wear an eye patch. Atropine is one of the oldest eye medications out there and has been used since Victorian times when it was used to dilate women's eyes to make them look more striking. It is extracted from the belladonna nightshade plant ... thus, comes the saying "belle of the ball." It is on the generic list at most pharmacies and is inexpensive.

Augmentin. An antibiotic pill that is good for skin, sinus, and inner-ear infections. It can cause mild diarrhea. Another oral medication I use is Keflex.

autorefractor. This is a machine used in the eye doctor's office to help determine your glasses prescription. While not as accurate as actual refraction (the process by which you read the eye chart through the phoropter machine), the autorefractor provides a useful starting point that can be further refined in the exam room.

Avastin. This is an injection medicine used to treat wet macular degeneration and sometimes used for other causes of macular edema such as diabetic retinopathy. Avastin was originally developed for systemic use to treat colon cancer. However, its anti-VEGF properties are good at targeting abnormal retinal blood vessels and so it is commonly used in the eye as well. Avastin is a wonder drug, and compared to comparable injectables (Lucentis, Macugen, Eylea), it is extremely cheap. The reason behind this cost is that Avastin was originally packaged in much larger dosage for systemic delivery for the entire body. Compounding pharmacies can split this large dosage into increments more suitable for ocular injection and the cost comes down to about 50 dollars a treatment. Compare this to medicines approved and marketed specifically for the eye which cost around $2,000 per treatment ... it makes you wonder how pharmaceuticals get away with it, huh?

AzaSite. This is an antibiotic drop containing azithromycin. You may know azithromycin in its pill form, where it is marketed as the "Z-pack" and is good for treating lung infections and pneumonia. AzaSite has been packaged as an eye drop and is sometimes used in treating blepharitis (chronic eyelid inflammation). The drop may have some anti-inflammatory properties, and it may help the eyelid meibomian glands flow better and improve eye comfort.

azithromycin. An antibiotic pill commonly used for pneumonia and upper respiratory infections. It is available as a dose pack called a "Z-pack." This medicine has been formulated into an eye drop called AzaSite for topical use for eye infection and for the treatment of blepharitis (chronic eyelid inflammation).

Azopt. A glaucoma eye drop used to lower eye pressure by slowing the production of aqueous fluid inside the eye. This is a carbonic anhydrase inhibitor. Other glaucoma drops in this class include Trusopt and dorzolamide.

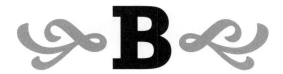

EYE CARTOON

by Tim Root, M.D.

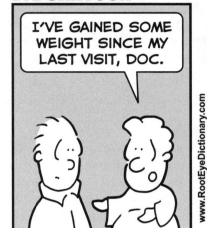

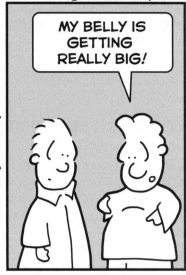

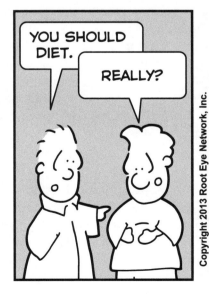

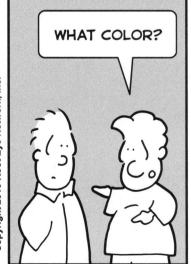

baby shampoo. A non-irritating shampoo sometimes used for treating blepharitis. Read the entry on lid scrubs for more details on how baby shampoo is used with the eyes.

bacitracin. An antibiotic used primarily for eye and skin infections. It is available as an ointment, and is found in other "combination" medications like neosporin and polysporin. Interesting tidbit about this drug: it was discovered at Columbia University (my alma mater) in 1943, and derived from a strain of Bacillus bacteria found in a 7-year-old girl named Margaret Tracy. The researchers therefore named the drug "bacitracin."

bacterial conjunctivitis. This is an infection in the eye involving the conjunctiva skin (the white of the eye). When it comes to conjunctivitis (also known as 'pink eye') it is often hard to determine the exact cause of an eye infection ... be it allergic, viral, or bacterial. Symptoms and presentation can give us clues, however. Bacterial infections typically involve only one eye and cause a purulent (pus) discharge. This discharge can be so bad that the eyelashes glue themselves shut in the morning. Treatment is with topical antibiotics. Mild to moderate cases may be amenable to ointments such as erythromycin, while severe cases may require multiple antibiotics. I also recommend people maintain good eyelid hygiene, cleaning the debris of their eyelashes with warm soapy water a few times a day (see lid scrubs). Also, wash your hands frequently as this eye infection could be contagious, though not nearly as contagious as viral conjunctivitis. As long as the vision is unaffected, bacterial conjunctivitis is rarely serious. Any red eye, however, needs to be evaluated to rule out more serious conditions like a corneal ulcer or uveitis.

BAK. This stands for benzalkonium chloride. BAK is a preservative found in many eye drops and rewetting drops. This preservative is necessary to keep bacteria from colonizing the bottle after being opened. Unfortunately, the preservative itself is a little harsh on the cornea. This is one of the reasons why we don't recommend using drops more than four times a day. This is particularly important for our dry eye and glaucoma patients who may be taking numerous eye medications.

Fortunately, there are now preservative-free rewetting drops available. Many of the glaucoma medications are now available in more expensive preservative-free versions (Zioptan and preservative-free Cosopt).

benzalkonium chloride. This is a preservative used in many eye drops to keep the bottles from being colonized from bacteria in the environment. See BAK for more information.

Bepreve. This is a prescription strength allergy drop. It is good for ocular itching and swelling around the eyes. It is usually dosed twice a day. This is one of my favorite drops and I have had good success with it. Similar prescription allergy drops include Pataday and Lastacaft.

Besivance. This is an antibiotic (besifloxacin) used with eye infections and after cataract surgery. This drug is in the fluoroquinolone class of drugs and is good for treating contact lens-related infections as well. The claim to fame with this particular medicine is that it was developed only for the eye and not used for systemic infections (or on chickens in poultry farms) so there is less chance of bacterial resistance developing. Comparable drops in the same drug class include Zymaxid (gatifloxacin) and Vigamox (moxifloxacin).

beta-carotene. This is the red-orange pigment found in carrots. It is converted to Vitamin A inside the body. Vitamin A is important in the retina for converting light into an electrical signal at the photoreceptors. High doses of Vitamin A have been used for the treatment of retinitis pigmentosa. This vitamin is also found in the eye vitamins used for the treatment of macular degeneration (see the AREDS Study for more information on this use). Beta-carotene is associated with increased rates of lung cancer in smokers, which is why smokers with macular degeneration need to make sure they read the contents of any eye vitamins they take. Smokers should also stop smoking ... but that goes without saying.

Betagan. This is a beta blocker eye drop used in the treatment of glaucoma. The generic name is levobunolol. I rarely prescribe this medication given the universal availability of timolol (which has the same efficacy and mechanism of action). Both of these drops are generic and inexpensive.

betaxolol. This is a selective beta-blocker eye drop used for treating glaucoma. This medication is similar to timolol, except it may have less systemic side effects such as bronchospasm (asthma). I don't prescribe this drop often, as betaxolol can be expensive and few of my patients complain of timolol side effects.

Betimol. A trade name for the glaucoma eye drop timolol. Timolol is a common beta-blocker glaucoma eye drop that has been around for a long time and is available in generic form.

Betoptic. This is the trade name for the drug betaxolol, a beta-blocker eye drop used for treating glaucoma. Unlike other beta-blockers (like timolol), this is a "selective" blocker with less systemic side effects. That being said, it is not often used because the side effects of timolol are usually negligible and timolol is available as an incredibly cheap generic.

bifocals. This is a secondary lens built into the bottom of glasses to help with reading. Though there is some historical debate, most people credit Benjamin Franklin as the inventor of the modern bifocal. There are many styles of modern bifocals. Progressive lenses are bifocals, without a visible line, that progress to a stronger view the further down the glass you look.

bimatoprost. This is the medication Lumigan, a prostaglandin eye drop used to treat glaucoma. It works by decreasing production of aqueous fluid inside the eye. This drug is also found in Latisse, a cosmetic drug used to make the eyelashes grow longer.

blepharitis. Blepharitis is a catchall term that means "eyelid inflammation." There are many causes of blepharitis, such as rosacea and sensitivity to environmental irritants. For most people, blepharitis is a self-limited condition that causes episodic eyelid irritation. Most people complain of red, watery eyes with a sandy or gritty sensation. The eyelids may look red and many people notice their eyelashes falling out. Treatment involves lid scrubs, warm compresses, and antibiotic/steroid medications to cool the eyes down. While not truly an infection or a "disease," blepharitis can be somewhat chronic and very annoying. The key is to find a combination of lid hygiene and medical treatment that keeps the eyes comfortable on a long-term basis.

blepharoplasty. A surgical procedure to remove excess skin (dermatochalasis) from above the eye. The excess skin is removed in the operating room and sewn up with a running baseball stitch. This running stitch is typically removed after a week.

Bleph-10. This is an antibiotic eye drop containing sulfacetamide at a concentration of 10%. This class of medication is often used for skin infections and to treat acne and rosacea. I rarely prescribe this eye drop because of the potential for sulfa allergy and the slew of alternative antibiotic options available today.

blind spot. The blind spot is an area in your vision where you can't see. Every eye has a small blind spot. This is due to where the optic nerve enters the back of the eye. At this insertion site, there are no retinal photoreceptors, so we don't detect light hitting this area of the retina. Fortunately, the blind spot doesn't cause problems because our other eye is able to cover this area and our brain has learned to ignore the discrepancy. Certain eye problems like glaucoma can enlarge the blind spot. You can detect your own blind spot ... try covering your left eye and hold up your right thumb at arms distance. Keep staring straight ahead, but slowly move your right arm outwards. When you are about 15 degrees out, the top of your thumb will disappear. Congratulations! You've found your "B-Spot!"

Blink. A popular brand of <u>rewetting drop</u> that is available over the counter. Competing brands include <u>Systane</u>, <u>Refresh</u> and <u>GenTeal</u>.

BRAO. This stands for Branch Retina Artery Occlusion. This is a blockage of a retinal artery in the back of the eye. The <u>retina</u> is very sensitive tissue. Without a constant supply of blood and oxygen from the retinal arteries, it quickly starves and dies. The cause of an arterial artery blockage can sometimes be seen (often a cholesterol plaque) during an exam. Unfortunately, there is little to be done other than evaluating embolic risk factors with heart and carotid scans. Retina specialists may perform a <u>fluorescein angiogram</u> to determine the site and extent of perfusion loss.

brimonidine. This is an eye drop used to treat <u>glaucoma</u>. The trade name for this medicine is <u>Alphagan</u>. A newer version is out now called <u>Alphagan P</u>. This eye drop is dosed twice a day.

Bromday. This is an <u>NSAID</u> anti-inflammatory eye drop. It is commonly used after <u>cataract surgery</u> to sooth the eye and decrease the chance of <u>macular edema</u>. Bromday contains <u>bromfenac</u> and its claim to fame is its once-a-day dosing.

bromfenac. This is an <u>NSAID</u> anti-inflammatory eye drop. It is usually known by the trade names <u>Bromday</u>. This drop is commonly used after <u>cataract surgery</u> to decrease the risk of <u>macular edema</u>.

BRVO. This stands for Branch Retina Vein Occlusion. This occurs when one of the veins leaving the eye becomes blocked. With this blockage, blood can't drain out of the retina, so it backs up into the retinal tissue instead. This causes swelling, then hemorrhage, with resulting vision loss. The amount of visual change is quite variable and depends upon where the blockage occurs. The occlusion eventually clears and the blood resorbs but sometimes <u>macular edema</u> can persist. This may need further treatment such as <u>anti-VEGF injections</u> (<u>Avastin</u>)

or <u>FLT</u> grid laser to reduce the swelling. <u>Neovascularization</u> can also occur after a BRVO, though we see this more with larger <u>CRVO</u>.

B-scan. A B-scan is a type of <u>ultrasound</u> of the eye, similar to a fetal ultrasound. This is usually required to evaluate the interior eye when our view is otherwise obscured. For example, if a person has a dense white <u>cataract</u>, it is impossible to detect a <u>retinal detachment</u> or tumor inside of the eye without this technology.

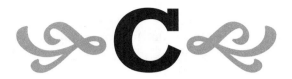

EYE CARTOON

by Tim Root, M.D.

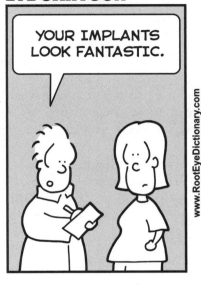

YOUR IMPLANTS LOOK FANTASTIC.

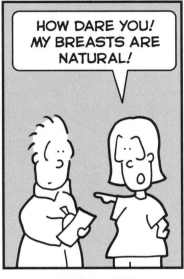

HOW DARE YOU! MY BREASTS ARE NATURAL!

www.RootEyeDictionary.com

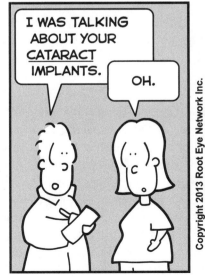

I WAS TALKING ABOUT YOUR <u>CATARACT</u> IMPLANTS.

OH.

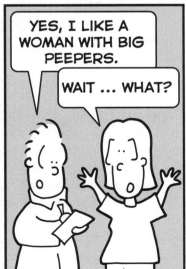

YES, I LIKE A WOMAN WITH BIG PEEPERS.

WAIT ... WHAT?

carbonic anhydrase inhibitor. This is a class of drugs that are often used for treating glaucoma. These drugs work by decreasing the production of aqueous fluid inside the eye. Examples of this drug class include Trusopt (dorzolamide), Azopt (brinzolamide) and the combination drop Cosopt. This medication is also available as a diuretic pill Diamox which we sometimes use for treating resistant glaucoma. Diamox also helps decrease intracranial pressure in cases of pseudotumor cerebri.

cataract. A cataract is when the normally clear lens inside the eye becomes cloudy. This cloudiness is a normal aging process and occurs in everyone with time, though congenital and premature cataracts can occur in youth as well. A cloudy cataract can cause visual difficulties. One of the earliest symptoms is glare or halos, especially with nighttime driving. Other symptoms include difficulty with fine visual details such as seeing distant road signs, reading small letters on television, and deciphering small print. As cataracts worsen, they can cause significant visual problems and even blindness. Fortunately, cataract surgery has advanced dramatically over the past few decades and cataracts are rarely a major problem these days.

cataract extraction. This is a fancy way to say cataract surgery. We say "extraction" because the cataract lens is removed from the eye during surgery. See cataract surgery for more details on the actual procedure.

cataract surgery. Cataract surgery is a procedure that involves removing the cloudy cataract from your eye and replacing it with a clear lens implant. This procedure takes only 15 minutes and with modern techniques can be done with no needles or stitches. A small microincision is created through the cornea to gain access to the cataract lens. The cataract is then vacuumed out using an ultrasonic probe. This is called phacoemulsification. A new intraocular lens (IOL) implant is then injected back into the eye. This implanted lens folds very small but once inside the eye, unfolds like a blossoming flower. This replaces your cataract with a new clear lens, improving vision and eliminating glare.

This is a high-tech, refined technique used by myself and most cataract surgeons due to its low rate of complication and rapid healing time.

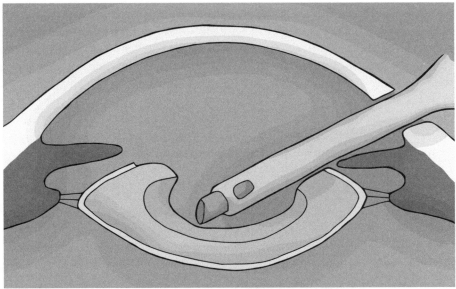

The cataract is vacuumed out with <u>phacoemulsification</u>

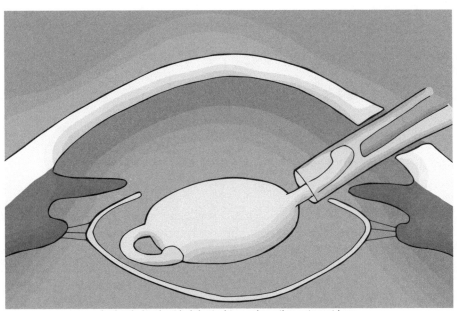

A plastic <u>implant</u> is injected to replace the <u>cataract</u> <u>lens</u>.

cellulitis. This is an infection of the skin around the eye. The cause for cellulitis is sometimes obvious - a scratch on the skin or bug bite becomes infected. Many times, however, the initial insult is not discovered. A cellulitis infection spreads under the skin and causes skin redness, heat, and impressive eyelid swelling. When isolated to the superficial layers of skin, this type of infection is generally minor and is treated with oral antibiotics and careful monitoring. If the infection penetrates deeper through the septum layer of the eyelid, than the eyeball and ocular muscles can be involved. This is called post-septal or "orbital" cellulitis. This deeper infection is serious and usually warrants hospitalization, IV antibiotics, and potentially, abscess drainage.

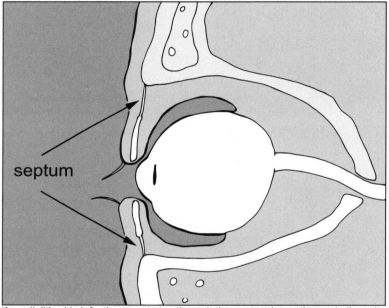

septum

If a cellulitis skin infection penetrates through the septum layer, the eyeball can be affected. The infection can even travel back toward the brain, so this is serious.

central retinal artery. This is the main artery that supplies blood to the eye, specifically the retina. The artery travels inside the optic nerve. Once the artery enters the back of the eye at the optic disk, it branches widely within the superficial layers of the retina. These coursing blood vessels can be examined during a dilated eye exam. This is the only artery in the body that is visible to the naked eye (i.e., not obscured by opaque skin). Some medical problems, like hypertension, can be detected by looking at this artery during an eye exam.

central retinal artery occlusion (CRAO).

This is a blockage of the all-important central retinal artery that supplies blood to the inner eye. This blockage usually occurs from embolic sources, such as a cholesterol plaque from the carotid artery or a blood clot from an irregular beating heart. Unfortunately, the retina has no backup blood supply, so when the central retinal artery is clogged, retinal damage occurs rapidly. Symptoms are usually described as a "blacking out" of the vision or seeing a "curtain coming down" associated with severe vision loss. This vision loss is usually permanent and treatment is usually focused on finding the cause to avoid future embolic problems that might cause more eye problems ... or even a stroke.

central retinal vein.

This is the main vein that drains blood out of the eye and away from the retina. This vein runs with the central retinal artery and leaves the eye through the optic nerve.

central retinal vein occlusion (CRVO).

This is a blockage of the main vein that drains blood out of the eye. Without this drainage, blood can't get out of the eye and it backs up into the retina. The retina can become swollen with blood, causing serious problems. Depending upon the severity of the swelling, vision can be severely affected, though it sometimes improves with time (though rarely as good as new). Treatment may involve a fluorescein angiogram to evaluate the extent of damage and sometimes laser therapy or anti-VEGF injections if there is residual retinal swelling. One potential problem after a CRVO is neovascularization ... this is the formation of abnormal blood vessels inside the eye that can cause future retinal damage and, if the new vessels block the angle, a severe angle closure glaucoma as well.

cephalexin.

An oral antibiotic (trade name Keflex) that is often used for skin and sinus infections. This pill is available as an inexpensive generic. Some people find it a little harsh on the stomach.

chalazion.

This is a large lump that forms in the eyelid. They occur when one of the oil-producing meibomian glands that run along the eyelid margin become blocked. Oil backs up into the eyelid, and causes a large bump ... this can be tender at first but usually becomes painless with time. Sometimes <u>warm compresses</u> and massage can make these chalazions drain away on their own. Often, however, an inflammatory "capsule" will form around the oil and the bump remains no matter how aggressive you are with massage. In these cases we can manually drain the chalazion. This involves numbing the skin with <u>lidocaine</u>, flipping the eyelid over, and draining the chalazion from the inside of the eyelid (to avoid scarring on the outer eyelid skin). This speeds recovery, but the chalazion can still take many months to go away completely.

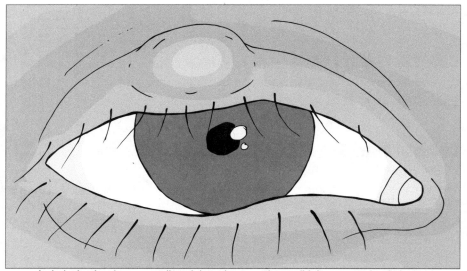

A chalazion is a large, usually painless, lump on the eyelid. It may require drainage.

chemical injury. A chemical splash to the eye can be very painful and potentially blinding. Strong acids and bases can cause <u>corneal</u> scarring and permanent vision loss if not treated promptly. The most common chemical injuries seen are from household cleaners splashed into the eye. Other toxins include hair dye, ear medicines, and anti-fungal nail drops mistakenly used in the eyes. The treatment for any chemical injury is irrigation - immediately wash the eye out. The faster and more thorough you wash your eye, the better the ultimate outcome. In the emergency room, doctors will occasionally use a Morgan lens, a plastic cup placed in the eye that is attached to bags of saline to allow copious irrigation over 15-30 minutes. Chemical splashes are the only eye problem where we recommend a therapy "before" you even see the doctor.

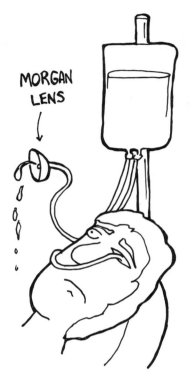

MORGAN LENS

chemosis. This is swelling of the <u>conjunctiva</u> skin, usually from allergy. The surface of the eye is covered by a very thin layer of skin called the conjunctiva. This skin layer is clear, but has blood vessels running through it that you can see when looking at the white of the eye in the mirror. Irritation to this skin causes fluid to collect under the surface and bulge this skin forward. This swelling can be quite impressive and alarming. As long as the vision is unchanged, however, this is rarely an emergency. Treatment usually involves <u>allergy drops</u> and occasionally <u>steroid</u> eye drops to decrease swelling.

choroid. The choroid is a layer of blood vessels that lie underneath the <u>retina</u> and supply some of the blood supply to the retina. The choroid circulation also helps remove the waste products from the <u>photoreceptors</u> (<u>rods</u> and <u>cones</u>) and processes them back into the circulatory system. Conditions like macular degeneration create a blockage between the choroid and retina, leading to retinal atrophy over time and vision loss.

chronic open angle glaucoma. This is the most common type of glaucoma. Glaucoma is usually described as high pressure inside the eye that causes damage to the optic nerve over time. The mechanism of this damage is not entirely clear ... but something about high pressure causes atrophy of the optic nerve over many years. The optic nerve is important because it connects the eyeball to the brain, and when damaged, the vision is permanently damaged. Most people with glaucoma have the "chronic open angle" variety, which is also called primary open angle glaucoma (POAG) or just plain "glaucoma." It is believed that something microscopic clogs the drainage "filter" inside the eye, leading to chronically elevated pressure. Unfortunately, there is no single test to determine if someone has glaucoma, so we look at several risk factors to determine risk and monitor progress. This includes eye pressure (obviously), visual fields (to evaluate peripheral vision), and OCT photographs of the optic nerve looking for changes that might indicate progression. Treatment is geared toward lowering the eye pressure with medication eye drops, laser therapies (SLT), and even surgery in advanced cases.

ciliary body. This is a ring of muscle that sits behind the iris (the colored part of the eye). The ciliary body has two main functions - to focus the vision and to produce aqueous fluid. To help the eye focus, the ciliary muscle can contract like a sphincter. The ciliary body is attached to the lens by zonules (strings) in a 360-degree ring (like the springs on a trampoline). When the ciliary muscle contracts, the tension on the zonular springs relaxes and the lens changes shape accordingly. This helps focus the eye to see near objects. The ciliary body also has cells that produce the aqueous fluid that fills the front chambers of the eye. The production (and drainage) of this aqueous fluid is what determines the internal ocular pressure of the eye, which is important in our discussion of glaucoma.

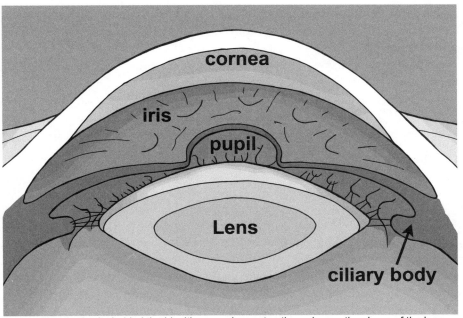

The ciliary body sits behind the iris. It's muscular contractions change the shape of the lens.

Ciloxan.　This is the trade name for the <u>antibiotic</u> eye drop <u>ciprofloxacin</u> (commonly called "Cipro"). Ciprofloxacin is a <u>fluoroquinolone</u> antibiotic that has good general bacterial coverage and is good for infections of the <u>cornea</u>. It may not be as powerful as the newer (and more expensive) medicines in the same class, however, such as <u>moxifloxacin</u> (<u>Vigamox</u>) and <u>gatifloxacin</u> (<u>Zymaxid</u>).

ciprofloxacin.　This is an <u>antibiotic</u> eye drop that is also available in pill form - it is commonly called "cipro." This antibiotic is in the <u>fluoroquinolone</u> class of drugs and therefore has good general bacterial coverage ... including covering most strains of <u>pseudomonas</u> (a particularly virulent bacteria found with many contact lens). Newer medicines in this class include <u>moxifloxacin</u> (<u>Vigamox</u> or <u>Moxeza</u>), <u>gatifloxacin</u> (<u>Zymaxid</u>) and <u>Besivance</u>.

color blindness.　This is when a person has a difficult time with color vision. <u>Cones</u> are the light receptors in our eyes that detect color and there are three types: red, green, and blue detectors. If any of these color-sensors are abnormal, color-detection will become flawed and a person may be considered "color blind." Many of the genes that control the development of these color cone cells are located on the X-chromosome. Males, who have only one X-chromosome to rely on, are more likely to have developmental color problems. In fact, about 8% of men have some color issues (usually difficulty with subtle red-green hues) while only 0.4% of women have this problem. There are a few conditions that can affect color as well, such as an active bout of optic neuritis and long-term use of the arthritis medication Plaquenil (though this is rare).

Combigan.
This is a combination glaucoma drop. It contains brimonidine (i.e., Alphagan) and the beta-blocker timolol. This drop is usually used twice a day. Combination drops like this decrease the number of drops you have to take and tends to improve eye comfort by minimizing exposure to preservatives like BAK. This convenience *may* cost more, however, as both brimonidine and timolol are available as generics when bought and used separately.

cone.
Cones are the photoreceptor in our retina that let us see in color. Cone cells are located deep in our retina and come in three different varieties, each sensitive to a different color spectra: red, green, and blue. Cones are very important for daylight vision and also for detecting fine visual needed to read small print. The macula, the central part of the retina that's responsible for our fine vision, is composed primarily of cones with more rods located in the peripheral retina. People with color blindness typically have a genetic problem with one of their cone types.

conjunctiva.
This is the thin layer of skin that covers the white part (the sclera) of the eyeball. The conjunctiva is very thin and has blood vessels coursing through it that you can see when looking in the mirror. The conjunctival skin also loops over and forms the inside of the eyelids themselves. This "looping" is what keeps objects like eyelashes and contact lenses from slipping completely behind the eye. When irritated, the conjunctival blood vessels dilate and make the eye look "pink." This is called pink-eye, or more formally conjunctivitis. If a blood vessel

breaks, blood can collect under the conjunctival skin and cause an impressive <u>subconjunctival hemorrhage</u>.

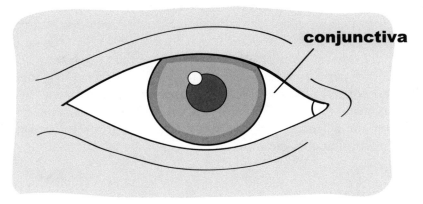

conjunctivitis. This is an irritation or infection of <u>conjunctiva</u> and is sometimes called "pink eye." There are many causes for conjunctivitis, but these usually fall into three categories: allergic, bacterial, and viral infection. With <u>allergic conjunctivitis</u>, the eye is typically irritated and "itchy." The eyelids can become puffy, and fluid can collect under the conjunctival skin and bulge it outwards (which looks quite scary). <u>Viral conjunctivitis</u> is what we usually think of as "<u>pink eye</u>." This is a viral infection of the eye similar to the common cold. Just like a cold, there is no effective treatment other than symptomatic relief and careful hygiene (as viral infections are quite contagious). <u>Bacterial conjunctivitis</u> usually affects only one eye and is associated with purulent (gunk or pus) discharge. This is treated with <u>antibiotic</u> drops. It is often hard (even for the eye doctor) to determine the exact cause of a conjunctivitis. If your eye is red you should see your eye doctor, especially if there is any change to the vision.

contacts. Contacts are plastic lenses that are placed directly onto the eye to improve vision. There are two main varieties: soft contact lenses, and hard rigid gas permeable (RGP) lenses. Most people use soft contacts as they are more comfortable and inexpensive, though hard RGP contacts are easier to manipulate with the fingers and get into the eye. Soft contacts have gotten so cheap that they are now available in disposable form and no longer require the extensive cleaning regimens of the past. Advanced <u>toric contacts</u> can now fix <u>astigmatism</u> and <u>multifocal</u>

contacts can sometimes help with reading vision. Colored contacts have color pigment silk-screened on the plastic to change eye color - I don't recommend these as they have a high rate of eye infection. The newer contact lens designs allow much more oxygen to permeate through the plastic and have been approved for extended wear so that you can sleep in them ... I don't necessarily recommend this either, as wearing contacts for extended periods dramatically increases the likelihood of infection, GPC, and corneal ulcers. Contact lenses are much harder to "fit" than glasses as they come in different steepness and diameters, thus contacts usually require a "fitting" for the first-time user and a refitting with any major prescription changes.

convergence. This is when the eyes turn inwards. For example, the eyes need to converge when looking at close objects such as when reading a book. People with a convergence insufficiency have a hard time with this and may have double vision when reading. Treatment may involve prism reading glasses and occasionally eye exercises to strengthen the inner eye muscles.

cornea. The cornea is the clear window in the front of our eye that lets light inside. If you were to touch the "colored part of your eye" with your finger, you'd be touching the cornea. The cornea is an extremely important part of vision - it acts as a fixed lens and actually provides the majority of the focusing power of the eye. Opacities of the cornea, from past infections or trauma, can severely limit fine visual acuity. The cornea has 5 distinct structural layers. The surface layer is called the epithelium. This layer is very thin and can scratch off if a foreign body gets in the eye. This is called a corneal abrasion. The middle layer is called the stroma - if an injury gets into this middle layer, scarring can form with possible visual consequences. The inside layer of the cornea is very thin and called the endothelium. This inner layer is important as the cells in this layer contain "pumps" that suck fluid out of the cornea. The cornea is clear because it is relatively dehydrated compared to other tissues in the body. If the pump mechanism of the inner cornea is injured or abnormal (such as in Fuchs' dystrophy or after a traumatic cataract surgery) the cornea can become too wet and cloudy.

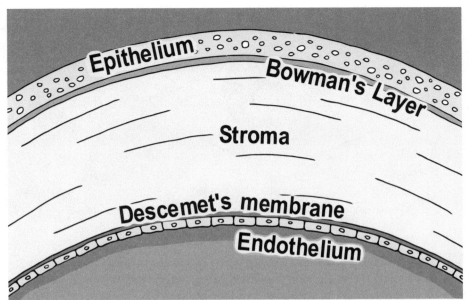

The cornea is made of five distinct layers. The outer epithelium is easily scratched off (corneal abrasion). The inner endothelium layer works like a pump to keep the cornea dry (see Fuchs' Dystrophy).

corneal abrasion. A corneal abrasion occurs when the surface layer of the <u>cornea</u> (the clear tissue that covers our eye) gets scratched. This usually occurs when a <u>foreign body</u>, like a piece of sand, gets into the eye. The surface layer of the eye is extremely thin and scratches easily. Fortunately, this tissue also heals quickly and most abrasions heal within a few days. Unfortunately, this process can be painful as there are more nerve endings in the cornea than anywhere else in the body. Treatment is usually geared toward avoiding infection with <u>antibiotics</u>. If the abrasion is large, painful, or healing slowly, other treatments may be instituted like <u>patching</u> the eye closed or putting a "bandage" contact lens on the eye. When an abrasion becomes infected, we call this a <u>corneal ulcer</u>. Most abrasions heal with no long-term consequences.

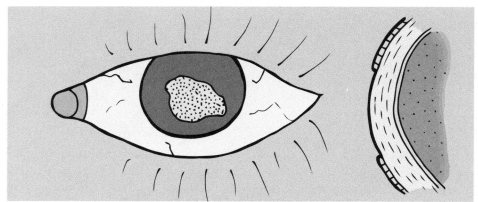
Only the superficial layer of the cornea is involved with a corneal abrasion.

corneal thickness.

The <u>cornea</u> is the clear window that makes up the front of the eye. It has a normal thickness of 540 microns and this can be measured in the office with a handheld device called a pachymeter (see <u>pachymetry</u>). Corneal thickness is important for a couple of reasons. When we check eye <u>pressure</u> using <u>applanation tonometry</u> (the blue light on the <u>slit-lamp microscope</u>) we press on the eye to measure how "hard" the cornea "feels." A thick cornea can give a falsely high pressure reading while a thin cornea can give a falsely low pressure. Thin corneas have been found to be an independent risk factor for <u>glaucoma</u>. Also, if you are contemplating <u>LASIK</u> surgery, you need to have a thick enough cornea to be a good candidate.

corneal topography.

This is the measurement of the surface characteristics of the <u>cornea</u>. See <u>topography</u> for more information on this topic.

corneal transplant.

A corneal transplant is when part of the <u>cornea</u> is replaced surgically. This may be necessary because of corneal opacities from past infections, traumatic scars, or decompensation of the cornea from prior intraocular surgeries. Several congenital abnormalities, such as <u>keratoconus</u>, may also need a corneal transplant to rehabilitate vision. Traditionally, a full thickness corneal transplant involves removing the central cornea and replacing it with a donor corneal button. This is done with extremely small stitches under a surgical microscope. These stitches are usually removed one by one over time. Certain conditions, such as <u>Fuchs' Dystrophy</u>, require only partial corneal transplants (called a <u>DSEK</u>) and have a much faster healing time. Because of advances in <u>contacts</u> and <u>cataract surgery</u>, corneal transplants are done much less often these days. This type of surgery is usually performed by a corneal specialist.

corneal ulcer. This is when an infection (bacterial, fungal, or viral) invades the <u>cornea</u>, the normally clear window that makes up the front of your eye. The cornea is unique because it is one of the few tissues in the eye that is clear, allowing us to see bacterial infections with no opaque skin blocking our view. Corneal ulcers usually look like a small white spot on the surface of the eye, though they are usually so small that they can only be seen using the <u>slit lamp microscope</u>. These infections can occur after a <u>corneal abrasion</u>, with <u>contact</u> lens use, and sometimes randomly with no obvious cause. Treatment is aggressive and involves <u>antibiotic</u> drops (often multiple antibiotics) to nip the infection in the bud as quickly as possible. Ulcers can be severe and penetrate all the way through the cornea and result in loss of the eye (very rare). Ulcers can also create scarring of the normally clear cornea. This scarring can limit the vision and necessitate a <u>corneal transplant</u> if severe enough.

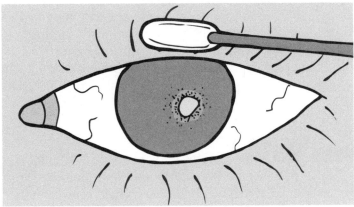
A corneal ulcer looks like white spot on the cornea.

Cosopt. This is a combination <u>glaucoma</u> drop. It contains <u>dorzolamide</u> (Trusopt) and <u>timolol</u>. It is usually used twice a day. A preservative-free version is now available, though it is more expensive.

cranial nerve palsy. The head and face are innervated by twelve separate "cranial" nerves. Each of these nerves has a different function. For example, the first cranial nerve (CN1) controls smell, while the eighth nerve (CN8) controls hearing. The main nerve we are concerned with is the second nerve (CN2) which is the optic nerve and transmits visual signals to the brain. The other nerves we watch are the ones that control eye movement ... this is the third (CN3), fourth (CN4) and sixth (CN6) nerves. If these "motility nerves" become damaged we call this a "palsy." Most cranial nerve palsies occur because of vasculopathic problems like diabetes or hypertension where the nerve doesn't get enough oxygen and shuts down. This is usually temporary and improves over six months. Other causes are more concerning, such as a tumor or aneurysm pushing on the nerve. See the entries on third nerve palsy, fourth nerve palsy, and sixth nerve palsy for more information.

cromolyn. An older allergy drop. I never prescribe cromolyn given the plethora of newer allergy drops available.

cross-eyed. This is when the eyes turn inwards toward the nose. In medical circles, we call this esotropia. This alignment problem can be congenital or arise in adulthood from a cranial nerve palsy or a stroke. In childhood, crossed eyes are usually corrected with strabismus surgery. The goal is to straighten the eyes for primary vision (when looking straight ahead and reading) to help with stereoscopic vision and avoid the formation of amblyopia. Prism glasses can also help alleviate double vision.

Crystalens. This is a premium implant used in cataract surgery that allows people to focus at both distance and near. Standard implants are fixed focus lenses, like a magnifying glass, and are only calibrated for one distance (i.e., you will need reading glasses after surgery). The Crystalens has a unique hinge design that allows it to rotate forward and back ... kind of how a telescope focuses. This more closely simulates the action of the original lens inside our eye and may eliminate your need for reading glasses after surgery. The effect of the Crystalens has had mixed results ... many people have good focal range afterwards, but others have much less effect (or the bifocal effect goes away after a few years). The nice thing about this lens, however, is that even if the bifocal effect doesn't work or wears off, the lens itself is just as clear as a standard lens implant and so no loss of actual "acuity" or "crispness" is suffered by choosing this lens. We are currently using more Restor lenses in our own practice, however, as the bifocal effect seems to be a little more predictable. Florence Henderson (the mother on the old Brady Bunch TV program) had a Crystalens for her own eye surgery and is featured in some of their commercials.

cyclopentolate. This is a moderate strength dilating drop used in the office to enlarge the pupils. This dilating drop lasts longer than tropicamide and is usually reserved for dilating children as they have strong eye muscles and are harder to dilate. This drop also has cycloplegia effects and is helpful when performing cycloplegic refraction in children. I occasionally prescribe cyclopentolate to help with photophobia (eye pain) for people with internal eye inflammation, such as from iritis or uveitis.

cycloplegia. This is when the eyes are dilated using eye drops. Certain dilating drops make the pupil larger, but they also paralyze the muscles inside the eye that control lens focusing. This paralysis is called cycloplegia. This effect is helpful when checking the vision in children (we call this cycloplegic refraction) as kids tend to "strain" when reading the eye chart. Eliminating this strain through temporary "cycloplegic paralysis" gives a more accurate prescription. Cycloplegia can also be helpful for pain control in people with ocular inflammation, such as iritis or uveitis. By paralyzing the muscles inside the eye, they don't spasm as much around bright lights, which makes the eye more comfortable overall. The cycloplegic drops we use in our office include tropicamide (most adults) and cyclopentolate (children). Atropine is the longest acting cycloplegic and was originally obtained from the belladonna nightshade plant - it was used in Victorian times to make women look "beautiful" by dilating their eyes. Most people have difficulty reading while dilated with cycloplegia drops.

cycloplegic refraction. This is the method for checking glasses prescription in children. Children have strong muscles inside their eye

that make it hard to measure their vision during a <u>refraction</u>. They can "strain" while reading the eye chart, throwing off our measurements. By using <u>cycloplegia</u> dilation drops, we temporarily paralyze these eye muscles and can capture a more accurate glasses check. Many children require their eyes to be dilated this way and this can really extend your office visit time tremendously.

D

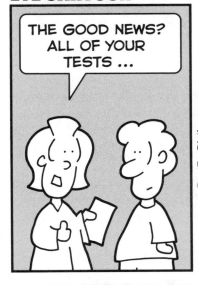

THE GOOD NEWS? ALL OF YOUR TESTS ...

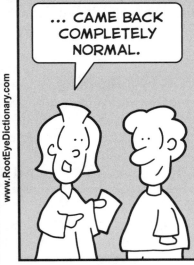

... CAME BACK COMPLETELY NORMAL.

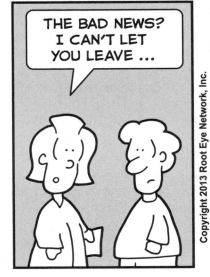

THE BAD NEWS? I CAN'T LET YOU LEAVE ...

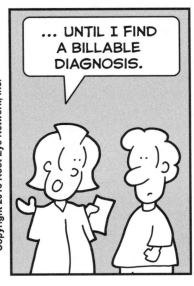

... UNTIL I FIND A BILLABLE DIAGNOSIS.

www.RootEyeDictionary.com

Copyright 2013 Root Eye Network, Inc.

dermatochalasis. This is excess skin that forms over the upper (and sometimes lower) eyelids. This skin can droop down to cover the upper eyelashes and even obstruct vision. If bad enough, a blepharoplasty surgery can be performed to surgically remove this skin.

dexamethasone. This is a steroid eye drop that is good at treating ocular inflammation. This medicine is normally found in combination eye drops like Tobradex (dexamethasone and tobramycin) and generic Maxitrol (dexamethasone, neomycin, and polymyxin).

diabetic retinopathy. The term diabetes is used to describe large amounts of sugar floating in your bloodstream. This sugar weakens the blood vessels throughout your body and makes them "leaky." This can cause health problems with major organs, including the eyes. For example, diabetics can develop kidney problems and difficulty with healing. In the eye, diabetic vessel leakage in the retina can affect the vision. The retina is the light-sensing structure inside the eye and can be compared to the film inside a camera. Just like camera film, the retina needs to be perfectly smooth and flat to take a good picture. Blood vessel leakage can make the retina swollen and lumpy. If this swelling occurs near the central visual area (i.e., macular edema) this can have severe visual consequences. Treatment in this case involves focal laser therapy (FLT laser) with a laser to seal off leaky spots. Diabetic leakage can be so bad that the eye fills with blood. This is called a vitreous hemorrhage and may require surgery to remove the blood if it doesn't clear on its own. Finally, long-term diabetic retinopathy can starve the retina of oxygen and can lead to the formation of abnormal retinal blood vessels. This process is called neovascularization and is the most severe stage of diabetic eye disease. These abnormal vessels can bleed, cause traction retinal detachments, and even clog the "drain" inside the eye and create an intractable acute glaucoma. Most of these diabetic problems can be avoided by maintaining good glycemic control and by getting regular dilated eye exams. It's better to detect and treat diabetic retinopathy early before these problems get out of control.

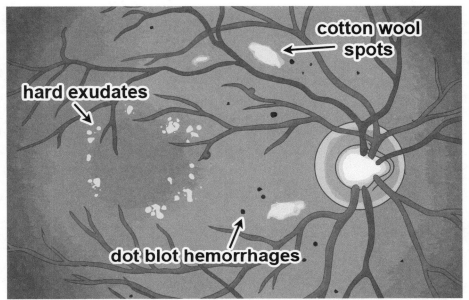

Diabetes can cause many retinal changes in the eye. These include micro-hemorrhages, macular swelling (with hard exudates), and nerve damage (cotton wool spots).

Diamox. This is the trade name for the oral medication <u>acetazolamide</u>. This is a water pill that is sometimes used in cases of poorly controlled <u>glaucoma</u> and to treat acute eye pressure spikes (such as after a complicated <u>cataract surgery</u>). Diamox can also decrease the pressure around the brain in cases of <u>pseudotumor cerebri</u>. See the entry on acetazolamide for more information.

diclofenac. This is an <u>NSAID</u> eye drop. Like all NSAIDs, diclofenac has a mechanism similar to Motrin or Advil and is good for inflammation. This class of medications is often used after <u>cataract surgery</u> to decrease the chance of retinal swelling (<u>macular edema</u>). This drop is also known under the trade name Voltaren. Diclofenac has gone generic, so it is much cheaper to obtain these days ... though most of my patients tell me it is pretty harsh going in.

dilated pupil. The <u>pupil</u> is the black "hole" in the middle of the <u>iris</u> (the colored part of the eye). The pupil looks black because the inside of the eye is dark. Eye doctors dilate the pupil with eye drops to help them view the retina. There are many causes for a dilated pupil outside of the doctors office, however. Some people have a natural <u>anisocoria</u> where one pupil is naturally larger than the other. Plant irritants, pesticides, and antihistamine medications can also make the pupil dilate. Blockage of sympathetic or parasympathetic nerves to the eye can cause a pupil to dilate - there are some serious medical conditions that can cause this blockage such as <u>Adie's pupil</u>, <u>Horner's Syndrome</u>, or <u>third nerve palsy</u>. A new onset pupil abnormality needs to be evaluated by an eye doctor.

diopter. A diopter is a unit of measurement that describes the power in a pair of <u>glasses</u> or <u>contacts</u>. For example, weak <u>reading glasses</u> have a diopter power of +1.00 while stronger readers have a power of +3.00 diopters. <u>Farsighted</u> people require positive (+) diopter glasses to improve their vision, while <u>nearsightedness</u> requires negative (-) diopter power. Many people have a small amount of <u>astigmatism</u> correction built into their <u>glasses prescription</u>, and this astigmatism correction is *also* measured in diopters. Finally, <u>prism</u> glasses are used to fix ocular alignment problems in people with <u>double vision</u> (for example, if you are <u>cross-eyed</u>). The amount of prism ground into a pair of spectacles is also measured in "prism diopters."

diplopia. This is when a person sees double ... that is to say, they see the same object twice. This can be a horizontal side-by-side doubling, a vertical up-down effect, or a combination of the two. Whenever a person has "<u>double vision</u>" the biggest question we ask is whether this is a monocular (one-eyed) diplopia or a binocular (two-eyed) problem. If the doubling goes away when covering either eye, then we know this is a binocular problem where the eyes are out of 'sync' with each other (such as with <u>crossed-eyes</u>). There are many

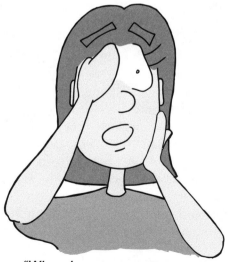

"When I cover one eye ... my double vision goes away!"

potential causes for binocular diplopia such as a <u>cranial nerve palsy</u> or a stroke. This alignment problem requires a thorough workup and may involve an MRI and neurologic evaluation depending upon our findings. If the double vision persists for many months, prism glasses or strabismus surgery may be required to get the eyes straightened out. Monocular (one-eye) diplopia is simpler and less concerning - if double vision remains, even when the other eye is covered, than we know the problem is located in *just* the eyeball itself. Monocular diplopia is rarely an emergency and can be caused by astigmatism, dry eye, cataracts, and rarely retinal problems like an epiretinal membrane.

dorzolamide

. A glaucoma eye drop used to lower eye pressure. The trade name is Trusopt but this medication has gone generic. This is a carbonic anhydrase inhibitor and works by decreasing the production of aqueous fluid inside the eye. It is usually taken twice a day. This medication is also found in the combination drop Cosopt (dorzolamide/timolol).

double vision

. This is also called diplopia, and describes the situation where you see the same object twice. This should not be confused with a ghost image where a dimmer "shadow image" is seen next to the primary object. See diplopia for more information on the causes of double vision.

doxycycline

. "Doxy" is an antibiotic pill that is often used in the treatment of blepharitis. With blepharitis (chronic eyelid irritation) one of the causes of eye irritation is from poor oil flow from the meibomian glands that run along the edge of the eyelids. Doxycycline has been found to help oil flow throughout the body, and this may help with the eye irritation. In fact, doxycycline is used for people with rosacea or acne because of a similar mechanism. This medicine shouldn't be used in children or when there is any potential for pregnancy. Also, it may interact with dairy products, and patients have an increased risk of sunburn while on it.

drusen. Drusen are deposits that form under the retina. They look like yellow spots in the retina and their presence is often a precursor to more serious macular degeneration. The retina is located in the back of the eye and functions like film in a camera. The retinal photoreceptors (rods and cones) are metabolically active and require a rich blood supply to function properly. Drusen are accumulations of "debris" that form under the retina, blocking the transfer of nutrients and oxygen between the retina and the supporting choroid (a bed of blood vessels that nourish the retina) underneath. This blockage of nutrition transport causes the retina to slowly atrophy and can lead to significant visual dysfunction over time. This process is called macular degeneration. "Macular drusen" should not be confused with optic nerve drusen which are calcium crystals in the optic disk that rarely cause visual problems.

dry eye. This describes ocular surface irritation that occurs from an irregularity of the tear film. Dry eye causes eye irritation and redness. Many people complain of a feeling that the eyes are "tired," especially in the evenings and when doing activities that require concentration (like reading, driving, or watching TV). Ironically, most people with dry eye complain that their eyes are actually watery. This is because dry eyes tend to sting. This irritation causes a tearing reflex from the lacrimal gland that overloads the eye with fluid. For most people, dry eye happens either because of an insufficiency in the *amount* of tears produced, or a problem with the *quality* of the tears produced. Treatment usually begins with over-the-counter rewetting drops. Other treatments include warm compresses (to open the tear glands), nighttime rewetting gels (to moisten the eyes while sleeping), punctal plugs (to keep the tears from draining too quickly), and medications such as Restasis. While dry eye sounds like a simple problem, it can be quite challenging to treat as it tends to be chronic and many of the treatments are short-lived.

dry macular degeneration. Macular degeneration is a progressive aging change to the retina where the retina seems to "wear out" and atrophy with time. Most people have "dry" degeneration, where the retina atrophies very slowly over many years. Gradual loss of central vision causes people to complain of difficult time reading small letters or seeing distant road signs. About 10-15% of people with dry degeneration will go on to develop "wet" degeneration. Wet macular degeneration occurs when blood vessels under the retina actually start to leak blood and serum, leading to rapid and severe vision loss. Even though dry degeneration can cause significant vision loss given enough time, it is considered the safer type of macular degeneration as its progression is very slow.

DSEK. This stands for Descemet's Stripping Endothelial Keratoplasty. It is a "partial" corneal transplant surgery where only the inside layers of the cornea are replaced. This is a vast improvement over traditional full-thickness transplants, as the surgical and healing time are much shorter and this surgery eliminates much of the risk of more advanced transplants. This type of surgery is primarily used with Fuchs' dystrophy, a condition where the inner corneal "pump cells" are unable to keep the cornea clear and need to be replaced.

Durezol. This is a powerful steroid eye drop occasionally used after cataract surgery. The stuff seems to be more powerful than Pred Forte, so I use it primarily with internal ocular inflammation such as iritis or uveitis.

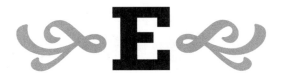

EYE CARTOON

by Tim Root, M.D.

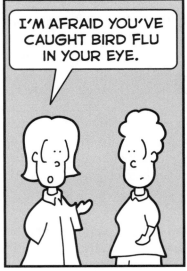

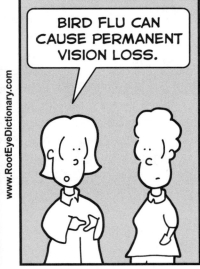

www.RootEyeDictionary.com

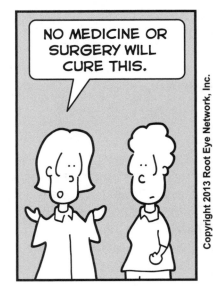

Copyright 2013 Root Eye Network, Inc.

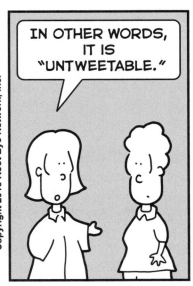

Econopred. This is a <u>steroid</u> eye drop that is commonly used after <u>cataract surgery</u> to cool down ocular inflammation. This medicine contains <u>prednisolone</u> acetate. Prednisolone is also available as a generic ... though there is some debate as to the quality of the generic steroid drop suspensions when compared to the brand names like Econopred and <u>Pred Forte</u>.

ectropion. This is an outward rotation of the lower <u>eyelid</u>, usually associated with laxity of the lower eyelid skin. This rotation causes the eyelid to pull away from the eyeball. This leads to <u>dry eye</u> and tearing problems. Mild cases can be treated with <u>artificial tears</u> and nighttime <u>rewetting ointments</u>. If the ectropion is bad enough, however, it may need to be corrected surgically, usually by tightening the eyelid to reapproximate its normal position. There are many causes of ectropion but the most common cause is simply skin laxity from age. The opposite of an ectropion would be an <u>entropion</u> where the eyelid turns inward such that the eyelashes are rubbing against the eye.

Elestat. A prescription-strength <u>allergy drop</u> containing the antihistamine epinastine. It is useful for treating puffy eyelids and ocular itching. Similar prescription-strength allergy drops include <u>Bepreve</u>, <u>Pataday</u> and <u>Lastacaft</u>.

emmetropia. This describes an eye that is neither <u>nearsighted</u> nor <u>farsighted</u>. An emmetropic eye is perfectly in focus for distance and does not require <u>glasses</u> to see far away.

endophthalmitis. This is an infection that occurs inside the eyeball, usually after an eye surgery or penetrating trauma. Internal ocular infection is dangerous as the eye is essentially a "big ball of water" and can quickly turn into an abscess. The <u>vitreous</u> gel does not have a vigorous immune response so that bacteria can replicate at whim and without tissue in the way to slow down growth. You can compare the eye to a swimming pool ... when a pool starts to turn green, it can go bad very fast as the algae replicates and spreads within the water. <u>Endophthalmitis</u> infection is rare these days thanks to modern surgical methods and prophylactic <u>antibiotic</u> coverage. If we suspect an infection, however, this usually means a trip to see our <u>retinal specialist</u> colleagues for a tap and inject (remove a sample for culture and injection of antibiotics inside the eye). If enough pus forms inside the eye, a surgical <u>vitrectomy</u> may be required to clean it out.

entropion.

This is when the eyelids turn inwards such that the <u>eyelashes</u> are rubbing against the surface of the eye. The eyelashes irritate the <u>cornea</u> and can even cause <u>corneal abrasions</u> and scarring. With mild cases we treat with ointments and plucking the lashes. Definitive treatment is surgical with an attempt to rotate the eyelid into a more normal (and comfortable) position. The opposite of entropion would be an <u>ectropion</u>, where the eyelid rotates outward away from the eye.

epiretinal membrane.

This is a clear membrane that can form on the surface of the <u>retina</u> and usually occurs with aging (though sometimes after ocular trauma). These membranes are common and can be detected with a dilated eye exam ... they look like a shiny glistening sheen on the retinal surface. While usually innocuous, epiretinal membranes can sometimes cause visual problems from retinal distortion. The retina detects light in the back of the eye. Like film in a camera, the retina surface needs to be perfectly smooth and flat to see well. Epiretinal membranes can contract and constrict, tugging on the retina and making the surface wrinkled. This can seriously affect vision if this distortion occurs at the <u>macula</u> (the part of the retina responsible for our fine central vision). If bad enough, these membranes can even open a hole in the retina (see <u>macular hole</u>). The severity of an epiretinal membrane can be evaluated by tracking vision and scanning the retina with <u>OCT</u> photographs. Monitoring at home can be done with an <u>Amsler grid</u>. Treatment is primarily surgical (though newer injectable medicines are being studied that look promising). A <u>membrane peel</u> surgery can be performed by a <u>retinal specialist</u>. This involves peeling the membrane off the retinal surface, then injecting a gas bubble into the eye to help "smooth" the retina back into its normal configuration. This entity is also called "cellophane maculopathy" or "macular pucker."

epiphora. This is a fancy medical way of saying "watery eyes." There are several causes for epiphora, but oddly enough, watering eyes is usually caused by dry eye. When the eyes are dry, they tend to sting and cause reflexive tearing. Occasionally, epiphora occurs because of nasolacrimal duct obstruction. This is when the tear drainage pathway running to the nose becomes blocked.

erythromycin. A popular and commonly used antibiotic ointment for the eye. This ointment is commonly used for mild to moderate infections and cases of blepharitis (chronic eyelid inflammation). This ointment comes in tubes and is available as an inexpensive generic. This ointment can be rubbed into the eyelashes at night or squeezed into the eye itself as it is an excellent rewetting ointment in its own right.

esophoria. This is a tendency for the eyes to drift inwards (cross eyed). Many people are born with a tendency for the eyes to turn inwards but they build strong eye muscles in youth to offset this. With age, these muscles may weaken and the eyes may turn inwards again, causing intermittent or constant double vision. When the eyes consistently remain misaligned, this is then called an esotropia.

esotropia. This is when the eyes turn inwards (cross-eyed). Ocular alignment problems like this can develop from many sources such as congenital crossed-eyes (which is usually treated with strabismus surgery during childhood to straighten the eyes out). Crossed eyes can also occur from decompensation of a pre-existing esophoria (a natural tendency for the eyes to turn inward). Acute crossing can happen after a stroke or cranial nerve palsy ... new onset diplopia (double vision) needs to be evaluated by an eye doctor.

excimer laser. This is a laser used in LASIK surgery. The laser "beam" produced by this laser has a very short wavelength which is outside of the visible spectrum (so it can't be seen with the human eye). Rather than burning or cutting tissue, this laser produces such intense energy that it actually disrupts molecular bonds and essentially disintegrates tissue. This is useful in LASIK surgery where corneal tissue is ablated (disintegrated) off the surface of the eye and allowed to "blow away in the breeze" ... without causing burns or scars on the clear <u>cornea</u> underneath.

exophoria. This is a tendency for the eyes to drift or turn outwards from each other. If bad enough, this can turn into a true <u>exotropia</u> where the eyes *do* turn outwards, causing <u>diplopia</u> (double vision).

exotropia. This is when the eyes turn outwards from each other ... and is sometimes described as "wall eyed" (the opposite of <u>cross eyed</u>). This alignment problem can occur for many reasons. Some people have a pre-existing <u>exophoria</u> (a tendency for their eyes to turn outwards) since birth but have built up strong eye muscles to keep their eyes looking straight. Later in life, these muscles can weaken and the eyes can start to drift out and cause intermittent (or constant) <u>diplopia</u> (double vision). Strokes or <u>cranial nerve palsies</u> can also cause an exotropia. Alignment problems like this need to be evaluated by an eye doctor, especially if sudden onset. Treatment is first geared toward finding any underlying cause. Double vision may be treated with <u>prism</u> glasses, eye exercises, or even <u>strabismus surgery</u>.

extraocular muscles. These are the muscles that control eye movement. Eye muscles insert onto the sides of the eyeball and contract (shorten) to rotate the eye in different directions. Any problem with these extraocular muscles (such as a <u>cranial nerve palsy</u>) can make the eyes go out of alignment and cause double vision (<u>diplopia</u>). With <u>strabismus surgery</u> (surgery to straighten the eyes out) the extraocular muscles can be strengthened or weakened by shortening these muscles or by changing their insertion point on the eyeball. Medical conditions like <u>Graves' disease</u> and <u>myasthenia gravis</u> can also affect the function of the extraocular muscles and cause double vision.

eye chart. The chart used in an eye doctor's office to measure vision. See <u>Snellen chart</u>.

eyelash.   Eyelashes are the small hairs that grow from the eyelid margin that serve to protect the eyes from foreign bodies. The lashes also protect the eye by providing sensory information and activating the blink reflex when touched. Certain glaucoma medications (like latanoprost) can make the eyelashes grow thicker and longer. The medication Latisse can also make lashes longer and is sold specifically for this purpose. Trichiasis is the term used to describe abnormal eyelashes that grow in the wrong direction and rub against the eyeball. People can lose their lashes after chemotherapy and from chronic eyelid inflammation from blepharitis.

eyelid. The eyelid is the mobile tissue that covers the eye, protecting the ocular surface and aiding with lubrication. The eyelids have two distinct layers. The outer layer contains the surface skin and muscles (that function to close the eyes). The inner layer contains the tarsal plate - this is a thick layer with a consistency of cartilage that gives the lid its integrity. Eyelashes run along the lid margin and serve to protect the eye from foreign bodies Also running along the lid margin is a row of excretory pores called the meibomian glands. These glands produce oil which is an important component of the tear film. If these pores clog up, the oil can back up and turn into a chalazion. At the inner margin of the eyelids, near the nose, are two drainage holes called the punctum (see puncta).   These punctum drain excess tears into the nose via the nasolacrimal duct. With nasolacrimal duct obstruction, this drainage is blocked and leads to watery eyes. Tears are produced continuously by cells embedded in the eyelid and the surface of the conjunctiva of the eyeball itself. Extra "reflexive tearing" is produced by the lacrimal gland which is located underneath the upper eyelid.

eyelid fasciculation. This is a fancy way of saying "twitching eyelid." Fasciculations are quite common, with people complaining that their whole eye has been twitching and jumping. Upon further discussion, we discover that it is actually their eyelid that has been twitching ... they can both feel it, and often see the skin movement when looking in the mirror. These fasciculations are strange, but almost always harmless and usually caused by minor irritation to the eye. I like to compare eyelid twitching to hiccups. Hiccups usually start when water goes down the "wrong pipe." This creates a sensation that the body needs to cough or retch ... and yet, this body reaction is "overkill." Instead, a funny feedback loop forms between the throat and diaphragm and results in rhythmic hiccups. A similar process may occur with the eye. The ocular surface may be slightly irritated and the eye "thinks" it needs to blink. However, the irritation isn't really that bad, so the eyelid ends up twitching instead. The "eye hiccup" theory is my own, and while not entirely accurate, sums up the underlying process for most people. Most people get their lid twitching in waves, with them occurring off and on for several weeks then nothing for months. Certain stressors like caffeine, weather changes, and diet may set them off. If they are bothersome, I tell my patients to use artificial tears and antihistamine allergy drops. If the twitching involves the rest of the face and mouth (hemifacial spasm), occurs in both eyes at the same time (blepharospasm), or the vision itself "shakes" during the episodes (superior oblique myokymia) ... this is more concerning and you need to be evaluated with an eye exam and possibly a neurologic consult.

eye vitamins. Vitamin supplementation has been found to be beneficial for people with macular degeneration. A large clinical trial called the AREDS Study was sponsored by the National Eye Institute. Its purpose was to look for supplements that might slow the progression of macular degeneration. They found that vitamins A, C, and E (along with the minerals zinc and copper) seemed to have a statistically significant benefit when ingested in high quantities. People with mild and moderate macular degeneration were 25% less likely to progress to advanced disease while on this vitamin cocktail, as compared to people taking a placebo. A follow-up AREDS 2 Study has found more supplements that might help, such as the plant pigments lutein and zeaxanthin. Eye vitamins are available over-the-counter and come in a slew of names and combinations. The most popular are Ocuvite, PreserVision, and I-Caps.

Eylea. An injectable anti-VEGF medicine used primarily for treating wet macular degeneration. Other drugs with a similar action are the injection drugs Avastin and Lucentis.

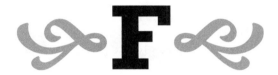

EYE CARTOON

by Tim Root, M.D.

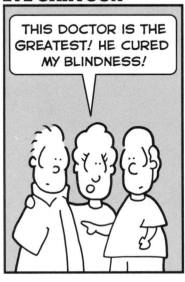

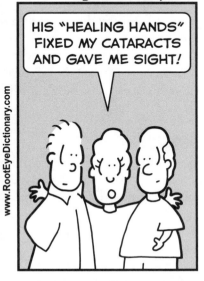

www.RootEyeDictionary.com

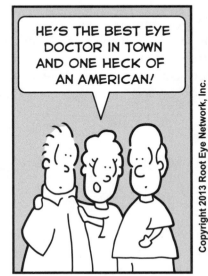

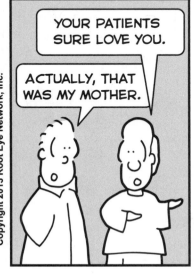

Copyright 2013 Root Eye Network, Inc.

farsightedness. This is a <u>refractive error</u> where close vision is blurry while distance vision is clearer. This situation occurs because the eye's focus is too "weak." Let me explain. Normally, the eye works like a camera with light entering the eye being focused perfectly on the <u>retina</u> - the retina is like the film in a camera, located in the back of the eye. When a person is farsighted, however, light wants to focus *behind* the retina and visual images look blurry. By strengthening the eye focusing power with glasses, light can focus properly on the retina. Many children are born slightly farsighted, yet still have excellent vision. This is because they have strong intraocular eye muscles that can change the shape of their <u>lens</u> (a process called <u>accommodation</u>) and see clearly. We lose this focal plasticity with age (a process called <u>presbyopia</u>) and most adults with farsightedness require glasses for BOTH distance and near vision.

femtosecond laser. A type of laser that delivers energy in super-fast spurts, coming out in rapid pulses like a miniature machine gun. This technology allows a laser to make finely controlled cuts in the <u>cornea</u> and helps in the creation of the "flap" during <u>LASIK</u> surgery - this is called <u>Intralase</u>. The femtosecond laser is occasionally used in <u>cataract surgery</u>, though its usefulness for intraocular surgery seems limited.

flashes. If you are seeing flashing lights in your vision, you are probably suffering from a <u>vitreous detachment</u>. This is when the <u>vitreous</u> jelly inside the eye contracts and peels off the <u>retina</u>. Many people describe seeing a flash like a "streak or arc of lightening" in their peripheral vision. While a vitreous detachment is relatively benign, those flashes can be the harbinger of more serious problems like a <u>retinal detachment</u>. Another cause for a "flash" is a <u>migraine aura</u> ... this is a special kind of headache that causes lights or waviness to the vision. These aren't truly flashes, however, as they usually persist for 15-30 minutes. New flashes warrant a dilated eye exam to rule out retinal problems.

flaxseed. Flaxseed and other plant-based foods contain omega-3 fatty acids that may be helpful in the treatment of <u>macular degeneration</u> (along with the heart benefits of the Omega-3 supplements). However, flaxseed contains mainly the ALA fatty acid ... not the EPA and DHA that are being studied in the AREDS2 Study. For the prevention of macular degeneration, traditional fish oils are probably better ... with flaxseed reserved for vegetarians and people allergic to fish. Those limitations aside, flaxseed fatty acids may be good for oil flow and so may be helpful for the meibomian gland dysfunction of blepharitis. Ground flaxseed is good; however, flaxseed oil can go rancid quickly (there is some question in the literature as to whether the *oil* can increase men's risk of prostate cancer).

FLT laser. This stands for Focal Laser Therapy and is the term used to describe most laser treatments used on the retina. For example, FLT laser can be used to seal leaking microaneurysms from diabetic retinopathy. Larger areas of retinal swelling and macular edema can be treated with FLT laser spots applied in a grid pattern to help peg the retina back into place. Small retinal tears can be isolated by sealing the surrounding retinal tissue with FLT laser spots - this keeps the tear from extending and turning into a retinal detachment. FLT laser spots are targeted to specific areas of the retina and is different than PRP (panretinal photocoagulation). With PRP, hundreds of laser spots are created throughout the entire peripheral retina in an attempt to save the central vision (typically used in cases of neovascularization from diabetic retinopathy or a CRVO).

floaters. These are little spots floating in the vision, which usually occur secondary to aging changes in the vitreous jelly that fills the eye. They are best seen when looking at plain surfaces like a blank wall or the sky and tend to move or "float" around with eye movements. While annoying, floaters are usually harmless. Sudden onset of floaters usually occurs from a vitreous detachment, which is a sudden contracture of the vitreous gel and is associated with aging. Floaters can also be a symptom of more serious problems like a vitreous hemorrhage or even a retinal detachment. New floaters need to be evaluated with a dilated eye exam to rule out serious pathology.

Flomax. This is the trade name for tamsulosin, an oral medication used for urinary problems in men with enlarged prostates. This medicine helps by relaxing smooth muscle in the urinary track, but it also relaxes

the smooth muscle in the iris, causing floppy iris syndrome. This creates challenges during cataract surgery.

floppy iris syndrome. This is an over-relaxation of the iris, usually caused by urinary medications like Flomax, that makes cataract surgery more difficult. The iris is the colored part of the eye - some people have blue irises and others have brown. The iris is a muscle as well, and this muscle makes your pupil large or small depending upon ambient lighting. Urinary medications like Flomax make your iris muscle "relax" and become "floppy." This relaxation can be so intense that when we make our initial microincision into the eye during surgery, the iris can bulge forward and actually block that incision! This makes surgery challenging, as you can imagine. There are many modern methods to deal with floppy iris ... but there is no doubt that Flomax makes cataract surgery difficult. This is especially true if your cataract is extremely dense or you don't dilate well. Floppy iris syndrome is something we see a lot in ophthalmology and the prevalence is increasing (Flomax has gone generic so we're seeing more usage). Other urinary drugs associated with floppy iris include Hytrin (terazosin), Cardura (doxazosin), and Uroxatral (alfuzosin).

fluorescein. This is a yellow dye used during an eye exam. This dye is an organic pigment similar to the pigments used in a highlighter ... at least in the sense that it glows under a blue or "black" light. This glowing property is useful for checking eye pressure during applanation tonometry. Fluorescein is also useful for detecting small scratches on the cornea (see corneal abrasion) or foreign bodies that are otherwise hard to see. These irritants may not be obvious to the doctor at first glance, but they glow brightly under the microscope with the help of fluorescein dye. Fluorescein is used for many applications outside of ophthalmology. For example, the yellow dye is used in bubble levels attached to work tools.

fluorescein angiogram. This is a diagnostic test performed by retina specialists to evaluate circulatory problems in the retina. Fluorescein is a harmless yellow dye that has the unique property that it glows under a blue/black light. This dye can be injected into the arm and introduced into the blood stream. As the dye works its way into the eye,

photographs of the retina are taken every few seconds to look for leaking areas or structural problems. This is particularly useful in detecting vessel leakage from <u>macular degeneration</u> and <u>diabetic retinopathy</u>, with the results helping to guide treatment. While this test is relatively innocuous, a small percentage of people have a temporary allergic reaction to the injection.

fluoroquinolone. This is a class of powerful <u>antibiotics</u> that is commonly used to treat eye infection and used as prophylactic treatment after <u>cataract surgery</u> to decrease the chance of <u>endophthalmitis</u>. These antibiotics are considered "broad spectrum" and are good for treating a myriad of different bacterial infections, including the dreaded <u>pseudomonas</u> infection common with <u>contact</u> lens wearers. Examples of second-generation fluoroquinolones are <u>ciprofloxacin</u> (a.k.a. "cipro") and <u>ofloxacin</u>. The newest generation of fluoroquinolones (<u>gatifloxacin</u>, <u>moxifloxacin</u>, and <u>besifloxacin</u>) are quite powerful and usually reserved for more serious infections such as a <u>corneal ulcer</u>. In the arsenal of available eye antibiotics, fluoroquinolones are generally considered the most powerful (and expensive). The only antibiotic more powerful would be specially prepared <u>fortified antibiotics</u> mixed up by a compounding pharmacy.

fluorometholone. A mild <u>steroid</u> eye drop. Also available under the trade name <u>FML</u>.

FML. Trade name for the drug <u>fluorometholone</u>. This is a mild <u>steroid</u> used to treat surface ocular inflammation.

foreign body. When a piece of dirt, plant, or metal gets into the eye, we call this a foreign body. Any foreign object in the eye will cause pain, watering, and occasionally an allergic response with swelling of the <u>conjunctiva</u> (the white part of the eye). Debris can scratch the <u>cornea</u>, causing further pain and increasing the chance of infection. The eye has more sensory nerve endings than anywhere else in the body ... even after a foreign body washes out, the eye can still hurt and feel as if there is something present. <u>Metal foreign bodies</u> are particularly nasty as metal pieces tend to stick to the cornea and rust into place. All foreign bodies need to be removed before the area becomes infected. This is done in the office at the slit lamp microscope using topical anesthesia drops - foreign body removal is a little nerve-wracking for the patient but surprisingly painless.

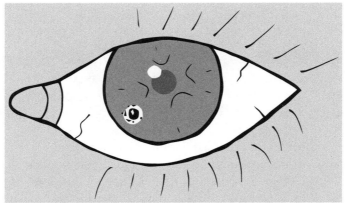

A foreign body can stick to the cornea and cause an infection or ulcer.

fortified antibiotics.

These are antibiotic eye drops especially made by a compounding pharmacy, used for bad eye infections such as a corneal ulcer. Certain strong medicines are not available in eye drop format (or don't come in high enough concentrations). If you have a bad corneal ulcer, for example, the typical antibiotic eye drops may not be strong enough. In these cases, we typically have a compounding pharmacy prepare fortified antibiotic drops. The most common drops we have created are vancomycin (an antibiotic good for MRSA), tobramycin (good general coverage), and amphotericin B (an antifungal agent).

fourth nerve palsy.

This is a paralysis or stroke to the fourth cranial nerve. This nerve controls a single eye muscle called the superior oblique muscle. This muscle is located behind the eyeball and it helps the eye look downward and assists with eye rotation when you tilt your head sideways. When the nerve is blocked, this muscle stops working, and people complain of vertical double vision where objects look stacked on top of each other. The double vision may get worse when looking to the side or trying to read a book. Fourth nerve palsies can be subtle. In fact, this is the hardest cranial nerve palsy to detect as the eyes appear normal to casual inspection. There are many causes for a 4th nerve palsy:

congenital, trauma, vascular insults (hypertension/diabetes), and lesions in the brain. If there isn't an obvious cause for a nerve palsy, then further imaging such as <u>MRI</u> should be obtained. If the double vision persists, <u>prism</u> glasses are an option as is <u>strabismus surgery</u>.

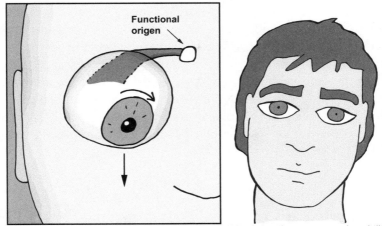

A fourth nerve palsy affects the superior oblique muscle, and can cause a head tilt.

fovea. This spot in the <u>retina</u> that is responsible for the *exact* center of our vision. The retina works like film in a camera and detects light. The most important part of the retina is the <u>macula</u>, which corresponds to our central vision. In the exact center of our macula is a small depression in the retina called the fovea. This is the most sensitive part of the entire retina and corresponds to your *extreme* central vision. For example, if you closely examine the period printed at the end of this sentence, the light bouncing off that period is focused directly onto your fovea. On a day-to-day basis, most eye doctors don't talk about the fovea but discuss the larger macular area in general. The fovea is more of an anatomical landmark seen on retinal scans like the <u>OCT</u> or <u>fluorescein angiogram</u>.

FreshKote. A prescription <u>rewetting drop</u> that contains several substances designed to replenish multiple layers of the <u>tear film</u>. It also has a higher osmotic (concentration) content than normal tears, which serves to help flatten the <u>cornea</u> cell layers and may be helpful for treating cloudy corneas (such as with <u>Fuchs' dystrophy</u> and <u>recurrent erosions</u>).

fresnel lens. A fresnel lens is a magnifying lens that is built into a flat piece of plastic. You may have seen fresnel magnifiers in a bookstore … they look like a clear, flexible sheet of plastic with tiny ridges along the surface. They are commonly used in overhead projectors and rear projection screen televisions. Fresnel lenses can be made very flat. Because of the many "ridge lines," they are not as clear as a normal lens, so they have limited use in eye care. The one exception is that a type of fresnel lens is used in multifocal <u>implants</u> like the <u>Restor lens</u>. This is a premium implant used in <u>cataract surgery</u> that has a <u>bifocal</u> built in. The implant has concentric rings built into its surface, with half the rings focused at distance and the other half focused for near. This technology can get people out of <u>reading glasses</u> after cataract surgery, though the fresnel effect can create visual side effects like ring halos and some loss of clarity.

fresnel stick-on prism. This is an adhesive <u>prism</u> that is stuck onto your <u>glasses</u> as a temporary method of fixing <u>double vision</u>. Prism glasses can be very effective for correcting alignment problems (<u>diplopia</u>). However, prism glasses are expensive and notoriously difficult to get made correctly. In some cases, I'll prescribe a temporary "stick-on" prism. It is a clear sticker, similar to a <u>fresnel lens</u>, that is cut out to the size of your glasses and adhered to the surface of the lens. This is cheaper then getting new glasses and allows you to see if you will tolerate the prism correction before more expensive prism glasses are made. The stick-on prism is somewhat unsightly, however, and not as clear as "normal glass" so is not a long-term solution.

Fuchs' Dystrophy. This is a condition where the cornea gets too wet and cloudy. The <u>cornea</u> (the clear window that makes up the front of the eye) is clear because it is relatively dehydrated compared to the rest of the eyeball. This may seem counterintuitive at first. After all, isn't the eye covered by tears on the outside and the inside of the eye filled with <u>aqueous</u> fluid? How can the cornea be dry? The cornea is dry because the innermost layer of the cornea has tiny cells that act like "bilge pumps," sucking water out of the cornea and continuously pumping that water back inside the eye. People with Fuchs' have less of these pump cells than normal and are at risk for their cornea getting too boggy and cloudy. This is especially true after eye surgery, as surgical trauma tends to shock a certain number of these pump cells so that they stop working. If the cornea gets wet enough to affect vision, then a corneal transplant may be needed. DSEK surgery is a newer type of transplant where only the inner layers of the cornea (including the pump layer) are replaced. Early treatments include hyperosmotic drops like Muro 128 and FreshKote. Glaucoma drops can help to lower the internal ocular pressure so that the pump cells don't have to work so hard.

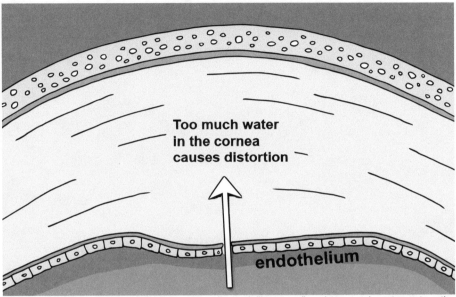

With Fuchs', the corneal endothelial pump cells can't "keep up," and too much water enters the cornea. This swelling distorts the cornea's anatomy and makes vision blurry.

fundus. This is another way of saying retina. The fundus describes the back portion of the retina that is visible using the eye microscope. For example, doctors use a "fundus camera" to take pictures of the retina. Fundus is a Latin term that means 'bottom' and is used to describe organ parts that look like the inside of a bowl. There is also a 'fundus' in the stomach, bladder, and in the uterus.

G

EYE CARTOON
by Tim Root, M.D.

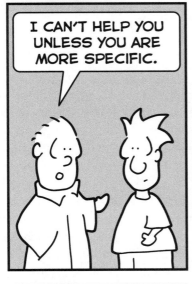

I CAN'T HELP YOU UNLESS YOU ARE MORE SPECIFIC.

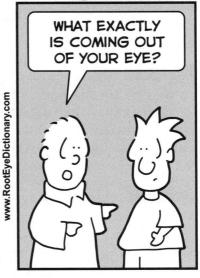

WHAT EXACTLY IS COMING OUT OF YOUR EYE?

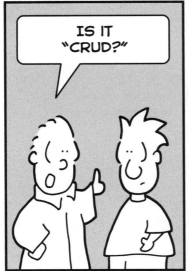

IS IT "CRUD?"

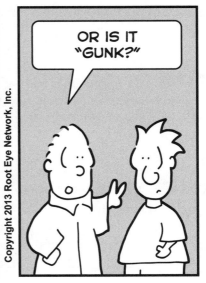

OR IS IT "GUNK?"

ganciclovir. This is a powerful antiviral medication that is now available as an eye ointment called <u>Zirgan</u>. We use this medicine in our practice to treat <u>herpetic eye disease</u>. <u>Retina specialists</u> occasionally use ganciclovir to treat viral infections (usually related to HIV) in the retina.

Garamycin. A trade name for the medication <u>gentamicin</u>. This is an <u>antibiotic</u> and is available as an ointment or eye drop. The generic equivalent is very cheap.

gatifloxacin. This is a powerful <u>fluoroquinolone</u> <u>antibiotic</u> eye drop, often used with more serious infections (such as <u>contact</u> lens related <u>corneal ulcers</u>) and after <u>cataract surgery</u>. The trade name for gatifloxacin is <u>Zymaxid</u>. Similar medicines in the same class include <u>moxifloxacin</u> (<u>Vigamox</u> & <u>Moxeza</u>) and besifloxacin (<u>Besivance</u>).

gentamicin. This is an older <u>antibiotic</u> eye drop that is also available as an ophthalmic ointment. This medicine has gone generic and is inexpensive, so I see it prescribed by many emergency rooms and urgent care clinics. While fairly effective, this medicine can be a little irritating to the eye with prolonged use. Alternative medicines like <u>tobramycin</u> drops or <u>erythromycin</u> ointment are also inexpensive and seem to be better tolerated.

GenTeal. A popular brand of over-the-counter <u>rewetting drops</u>. Genteal also makes a nighttime <u>rewetting ointment</u> called "GenTeal Gel" that is useful for extreme dry eyes. Competing brands include <u>Refresh</u> and <u>Systane</u>.

ghost image. This is when you see double, but the second image is less bright and usually offset to the side of the main object you are staring at. Ghost images are usually secondary to visual opacities such as a <u>cataract</u> or <u>astigmatism</u>. Upon further questioning, most people with monocular <u>diplopia</u> (<u>double vision</u> from a single eye) are often experiencing a ghost image or shadow rather than a true doubling of their vision.

glare. This is when you see halos or blur when exposed to bright lights. Many people with dense <u>cataracts</u> complain of glare while driving at night ... the headlights from oncoming traffic make it hard to see. Glare is usually associated with cataracts and one of the indicators that it may be time for <u>cataract surgery</u>. Another cause of glare is <u>corneal</u> swelling from diseases like <u>Fuchs' dystrophy</u>. Some people have sensitive eyes and seem to suffer from glare without any obvious anatomic abnormalities. Sunglasses during the day may help. At night, a glare-resistant coating on glasses may help.

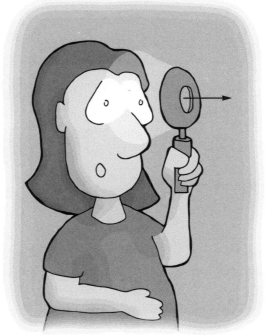

Glare problems can be simulated in the office using the BAT (brightness acuity test) device.

glasses. These are focusing lenses used to improve vision. There are many options when buying a modern set of glasses. For example, you can have them made with <u>bifocals</u>, <u>trifocals</u>, or even a no-line bifocal called a <u>progressive lens</u>. Glasses are also available as <u>transitional lenses</u> that darken when exposed to sunlight.

glasses prescription

glasses prescription. A glasses prescription is the little piece of paper that has your spectacle correction written on it. There are many numbers on a glasses prescription and they can be a little daunting to decode if you've never done this before. The first number is your basic refractive error: if you are farsighted this will be a positive number and if nearsighted this will be a negative number. The second number is how much astigmatism you have (if you have any). The last number is a degree measurement used to align the astigmatism glasses in their frames properly. Finally, the "add" is the power of any bifocal correction and can range anywhere from +1.00 to +3.50 depending upon your age and how close to your face you like to read books. OD stands for right eye and OS is the left eye.

Rx:

OD: - 2.00 + 1.00 x 180 deg

OS: - 1.50 + 0.75 x 020 deg

Bifocal Add: +3.00

glaucoma. Glaucoma is best described as high pressure in the eye that causes damage to the optic nerve. The optic nerve is the large nerve that sends visual information from the eye to the brain. High pressure causes damage to this nerve over time. Glaucoma is a very slow process that usually has no real symptoms other than peripheral vision loss that may go unnoticed until far advanced. Diagnosis is made by measuring the eye pressure, examining various risk factors such as family history and corneal thickness, and by measuring actual damage with optic nerve scans (such as OCT) and visual field testing. Treatment is focused on lowering eye pressure with topical eye drops, laser therapy (SLT), and even surgical treatment (trabeculoplasty or tube-shunt). Most people have chronic open-angle glaucoma and develop visual problems slowly over time. A minority suffer from acute glaucoma and develop acute pain, blurry vision, and extremely high eye pressure. If glaucoma goes unchecked, it will lead to permanent vision loss and even blindness.

glaucoma suspect. This is a person who "might" have glaucoma.

The diagnosis of glaucoma is not always an obvious one. There is no "one test" that says if a person has glaucoma. Instead, we look at various risk factors to decide if you look "suspicious enough" to have glaucoma. The most obvious risk factor is high eye pressure. If your pressure is "through the roof" ... then sure, you probably have glaucoma. The difficulty here is that "normal" eye pressure is different for everyone. Normal pressure ranges from 10 to 21. However, some people have pressures of 25 (or higher) and never develop glaucoma damage. Other people have pressures of 15 and yet are exquisitely sensitive to minor pressure elevations (this condition is referred to as low-tension glaucoma). Other risk factors we look at are family history and circulation problems like migraine headaches. A thin cornea, as measured by pachymetry, has been found to be an independent risk factor for glaucoma, though we don't know why. As glaucoma progresses, damage occurs at the optic nerve in the back of the eye and the optic disk begins to look hollowed out. This is called glaucomatous cupping. Your eye doctor can examine your nerves with a dilated eye exam and look for this appearance, but once again, some people have "suspicious looking nerves," but don't actually have true glaucoma. Finally, we can check for actual vision loss by performing a visual field. Glaucoma damage produces characteristic patterns of vision loss in your peripheral vision. Periodic eye exams are necessary to monitor for pressure fluctuations, photograph optic nerve appearance, and to detect visual field problems. This is all in an attempt to detect early glaucoma so that therapy can start, if needed.

glaucomatous cupping. This is a descriptive term for the

changes that occur at the optic nerve from glaucoma damage. The optic nerve is the big nerve that connects the eyeball to the brain. It is located at the back of the eye, and its insertion can be seen inside the eye in the retina. This nerve is like a tube or pipe, with over a million individual nerve cell "wires" running through it ... kind of like a bundle of wires running through a PVC pipe. With glaucoma, the nerve fibers die off one by one and eventually disappear. With time, this creates a hollowed out appearance to the optic nerve which can be seen during an exam. This hollowed out appearance looks like the inside of a bowl or "cup" and is called glaucomatous cupping. People with advanced glaucoma have significant cupping with hollowed out optic nerves. Some people have the appearance of glaucomatous cupping, but in reality have perfectly normal eyes. This is because some people are born with larger optic nerves ... their "pipe" is very large with a lot of excess room inside of it that gives the illusion of nerve loss, but in reality they are perfectly healthy. This anatomical variety is one of the reasons eye doctors take photos and scans of the optic nerve - to see if "cupping" has gotten worse over time.

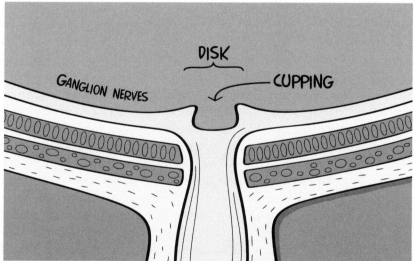

Glaucoma causes the nerves in the retina to slowly wither away. This creates a "cupped" or "hollowed out" appearance to the optic nerve (also called the optic disk).

gonioscopy. This is the eye exam technique used to examine the drainage angle inside the eye, and is used to evaluate for glaucoma. The front part of the eye is filled with a fluid called the aqueous humor. This fluid nourishes many structures inside the eye and the balance of aqueous production and drainage is what controls the overall pressure of the eye. The aqueous "drain" is called the trabecular meshwork and is located in a 360-degree ring ... right at the point where the iris (the colored part of the eye) intersects with the sclera (the white of the eye). This drainage intersection is also known as the "angle" because of the insertion anatomy. Some people are at risk for their angle to narrow and close, leading to complete blockage of the drain which causes an acute glaucoma. It is useful for an eye doctor to examine this angle in order to let their patients know their risk for having one of these glaucoma attacks. Unfortunately, the angle is a little difficult to see, even with a microscope, because of its interior location. Gonioscopy is the technique where a special lens containing mirrors (a goniolens) is placed onto the surface of the eye. The doctor then looks through this lens/mirror device to see how "open" the angle appears. If the angle seems very tight, the risk of an acute glaucoma attack is high, and a prophylactic LPI laser procedure can be performed to decrease this risk.

GPC. This stands for Giant Papillary Conjunctivitis and is sometimes called "contact lens overwear syndrome." Contacts are made of plastic, but at a microscopic level they look like a sponge full of water. Just like a sponge, contacts tend to suck up irritants from the environment. Contacts also block the amount of oxygen the cornea normally absorbs from the air around us. This combination of irritants can aggravate the ocular surface and create a temporary inflammatory reaction. The eye becomes irritated and intolerant to contact lens wear. On exam, the eye looks red and may even have focal spots of inflammation on the cornea itself. When the eyelids are flipped over, giant papillary "bumps" can be seen - they look similar to allergic hives that you get on the skin. GPC tends to occur more in people who wear their contacts for extended periods or who sleep in their contacts, though sometimes we see this in people who are very conscientious with their ocular hygiene. Treatment usually involves a contact lens "holiday" to let the eyes recover. Rewetting drops, allergy drops, and occasionally a mild steroid can speed the healing process. Hopefully, after a few weeks of rest, contacts can slowly be resumed.

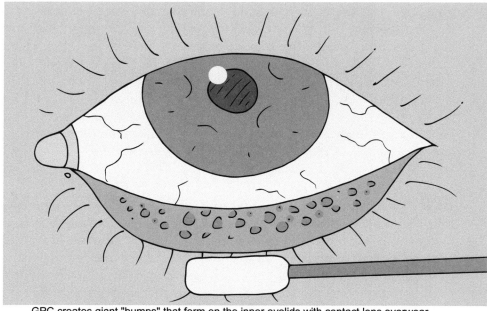

GPC creates giant "bumps" that form on the inner eyelids with contact lens overwear.

Graves' disease.

Graves' disease is an autoimmune disorder where the thyroid pumps out too much thyroid hormone. Graves' is the most common cause for hyperthyroidism and is more common with women. Graves' can cause ocular problems such as eyelid retraction (giving people a wide-eyed appearance) and swelling of the eye muscles located behind the eye. This swelling causes the eye to protrude forward - a condition called <u>proptosis</u> or exophthalmos. Protrusion can cause extreme <u>dry eye</u> and exposure problems if the eyelids don't close completely while sleeping. <u>Double vision</u> is common secondary to the eye muscle involvement. If bad enough, muscle swelling can push on the <u>optic nerve</u> behind the eye and create neurologic vision loss. Treatment is geared toward normalizing thyroid levels and lubricating the eye. If double vision is constant, <u>strabismus surgery</u> can be considered. Decompression surgery (usually with an ENT doctor or an oculoplastic surgeon) is sometimes performed to give the eye more room inside the eye socket.

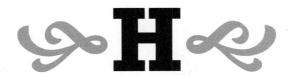

EYE CARTOON

by Tim Root, M.D.

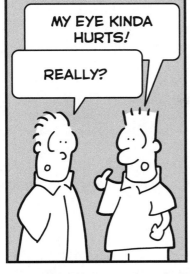

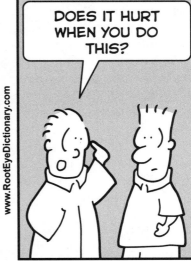

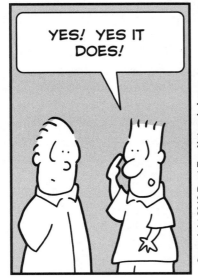

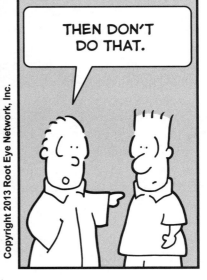

headaches

headaches. Headaches are common and their cause is difficult to ascertain. There are a couple of ocular conditions that can exacerbate headaches. If the eyes are out of alignment (a condition called strabismus) the constant eye muscle strain of looking straight ahead can cause a tension headache. Prism glasses or eye exercises may help with this. If the eyes have a refractive error (like nearsightedness or farsightedness) the strain of focusing can also cause a headache. Updating glasses or contacts may help in these cases. There is also a condition called pseudotumor cerebri that causes headaches because the fluid pressure inside the skull is too high. This disorder is hard to diagnose short of doing a spinal tap and measuring the "opening pressure" of fluid coming out. However, IF the intracranial pressure is high, fluid tends to travel up the optic nerve and swelling can be seen at the optic disk inside the eye during a dilated retina exam. Ocular migraines are headaches associated with visual changes or "auras" and are usually secondary to harmless spasms of blood vessels at the eye and brain. Finally, in elderly patients, headaches associated with scalp tenderness or general malaise (not feeling well) can occasionally be associated with a more serious condition called temporal arteritis, which may require oral steroids.

herpetic eye disease

herpetic eye disease. Herpes simplex virus (HSV) can cause cold sores around the mouth and can sometimes affect the eye. When the eye is involved we typically see a dendritic corneal ulcer on the surface of the eye. We call it "dendritic" because the infection forms a classic fern-leaf pattern on the cornea. Initial episodes cause eye irritation and a foreign body sensation, though repeat bouts are less painful due to viral deadening of the eye nerves. Deep and repeated infections can cause corneal scarring that may lead to permanent vision loss. The treatment for herpetic eye disease is usually a combination of topical antiviral drops such as Viroptic or Zirgan and an oral antiviral like acyclovir or Valtrex. Whenever we diagnose "herpes virus" in the eye, I like to stress to my patients that this is NOT a sexually transmitted disease that they've caught! These viral infections are almost always an activation of HSV-1 (the non-sexual variety of herpes). The majority of the U.S. population is seropositive for HSV-1 with the virus lying dormant in the base of nerves. Only in some people does the virus activate enough to cause skin and eye manifestations. The triggers for this are unknown, but there are many theories about emotional stress, hormones, or environmental conditions that might bring it out.

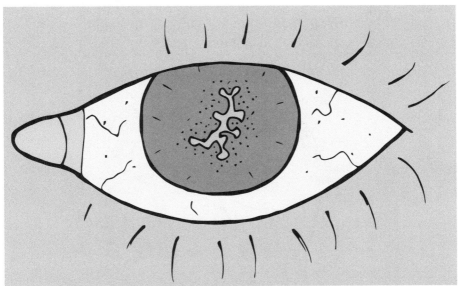

The classic dendritic ulcer on the surface of the cornea with herpetic infections.

homatropine. This is a long-acting dilating drop with <u>cycloplegia</u> effects. We sometimes use this to treat eye pain (<u>photophobia</u>), especially when the cause is internal ocular inflammation from <u>uveitis</u>.

Horner's syndrome. This is a <u>pupil</u> abnormality where the eye loses its sympathetic nervous system innervation. The sympathetic system helps the body function during stressful situations ... it is our "fight or flight" system. Sympathetic stimulation helps the heart beat faster and routes blood to the musculoskeletal system so we can run faster. In the eye, the sympathetic system makes the pupils dilate and the <u>eyelids</u> widen ... presumably so that we can see better in the dark as we run away from attacking grizzly bears. If the sympathetic connections to the eye are blocked, the pupil doesn't dilate well and the pupil looks small and constricted. Also, the eyelid droops a little (<u>ptosis</u>). The sympathetic nerves involved are very long, with a circuitous route from the brain, running down the neck, over the lung, and back up to the eyeball. Any obstruction in this pathway, such as a lung tumor, carotid artery dissection, or even a congenital malformation, can cause a Horner's pupil. This diagnosis is made in the office by examining the pupils in light and dark conditions. The location of the sympathetic nerve 'blockage' can sometimes be localized using stimulant eye drops. More imaging, like a CAT scan or <u>MRI</u> may be required if the cause for the Horner's is not immediately obvious.

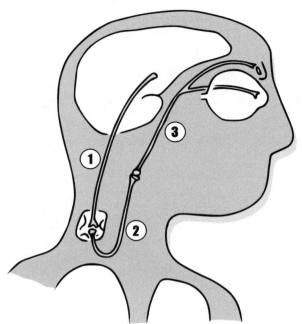

The sympathetic nerve pathway is long, and many dangerous conditions can occur along this route.

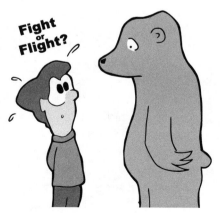

Sympathetic system helps our eyes dilate in stressful situations.

HRT. HRT stands for Heidelberg Retinal Tomograph ... but this is hard to pronounce so we just call it "HRT". This is an imaging test used primarily to photograph the optic disk in people with glaucoma. The HRT uses a scanning laser to create a three-dimensional map of the optic nerve that can be used to track glaucomatous cupping and detect nerve damage from advancing glaucoma. The laser photograph is painless and safe. HRT can also stand for "hormone replacement therapy" or "hostage rescue team."

HSV. This stands for herpes simplex virus and comes in two varieties. HSV-1 is usually considered the non-sexually transmitted herpes that causes cold sores. HSV-2 is the sexually transmitted variety that causes genital lesions. We typically see HSV-1 related infections when the virus activates in the eye. See herpetic eye disease for more information on this topic.

Humphrey visual field (HVF). A machine used to detect problems with peripheral vision. See visual field for more information on this common office test.

hyperopia. A fancy way of saying farsightedness. This means that you see far away better than close-up. See the entry on farsightedness for more details.

hyphema. This is bleeding inside the eye, occurring after trauma or spontaneously from neovascularization (abnormal blood vessels inside the eye). With a hyphema, blood leaks from internal blood vessels and pools in the front part of the eye (the anterior chamber). If there is enough blood, gravity causes the blood to sink into a visible 'layer.' A hyphema is easy to see under a microscope and can sometimes be detected with the naked eye. This is contrast to a vitreous hemorrhage in the back of the eye that can only be detected during a dilated eye exam. Blood cells can clog the aqueous "drain" and cause a temporary glaucoma, so treatment is geared toward lowering the eye pressure with glaucoma eye drops. Steroid drops are also used to decrease inflammation. Occasionally, dilating drops are used for pain control (a process called <u>cycloplegia</u>) and to keep the pupil edge from scarring down and forming <u>iris synechiae</u>. Hyphema bleeding usually occurs from a leaking blood vessel in the <u>iris</u>. A clot will form to stop this bleeding. After three to five days, however, this clot begins to break down and the eye is at risk for a 'rebleed.' For this reason, we will typically check the eye several times during the first week to monitor pressure and hyphema status. Anyone with enough trauma to cause a hyphema is at risk for developing <u>chronic open angle glaucoma</u> secondary to microscopic damage to the <u>trabecular meshwork</u> drain. After the eye has healed, we may look at this drain via <u>gonioscopy</u> to see if there is any obvious damage that can be seen.

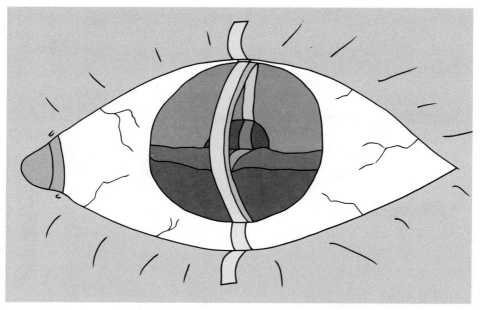

With a hyphema, blood can form in the anterior chamber of the eye and it tends to sink to the bottom and form a "layer" of blood.

I

EYE CARTOON
by Tim Root, M.D.

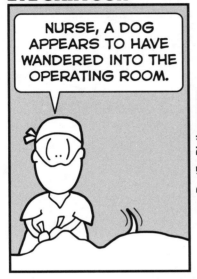

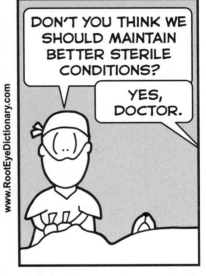

www.RootEyeDictionary.com

Copyright 2013 Root Eye Network, Inc.

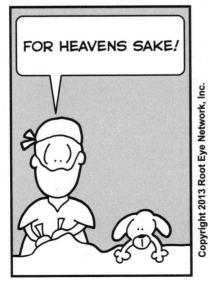

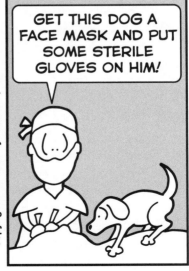

I-CAPS. This is one of the eye vitamins based on the <u>AREDS Study</u> used to decrease the rate of progression of <u>macular degeneration</u>. Just like the competing vitamin brands (<u>Ocuvite</u> and <u>PreserVision</u>) there are many variations in the formula. They appear to all follow the general AREDS formula, with several adding <u>lutein</u> and <u>omega-3</u>. If you are a smoker, look for a vitamin that doesn't contain <u>beta-carotene</u> ... beta-carotene is the precursor to Vitamin A and is thought to increase the risk of lung cancer in smokers.

ICG angiography. This is a type of angiography used by a <u>retina specialist</u> to look for problems in the <u>retina</u>. With this test, indocyanine green dye is injected into a blood vessel in the arm. As the dye travels through the circulatory system, it will eventually reach the eye's circulation. Photographs are then taken every few seconds to track how the dye flows and illuminates structures inside the eye. ICG is particularly good for examining deep structures in the retina, especially in cases of retinal bleeding where the view is otherwise obscured. <u>Fluorescein angiography</u> is a similar test, and more commonly performed. It looks for problems in the more superficial layers of the retina.

Ilevro. This is a new formulation of the anti-inflammatory eye drop <u>Nevanac</u>. This formulation contains three times the concentration of the drug <u>nepafenac</u>, allowing the medication to be dosed once a day. These <u>NSAID</u> eye drops are useful after <u>cataract surgery</u> to decrease the chance of <u>retina</u> swelling.

implant. This is a plastic lens that is placed inside the eye during <u>cataract surgery</u> and is sometimes called an IOL (intraocular lens). With cataract surgery, the natural <u>lens</u> inside the eye has become cloudy and needs to be removed. If a new lens is not put back in the eye, the vision will remain blurry and be completely out of focus. Before the invention of modern intraocular lenses, patients with no lenses (<u>aphakia</u>) had to wear "coke bottle" glasses just to see normally after their cataracts were removed. Modern implants are made of a flexible acrylic plastic that allows them to fold up very small like a burrito. This allows them to be injected into the eye through a very small incision through the <u>cornea</u>.

Once inside the eye, the intraocular lens opens up like a blossoming flower into its normal shape. Newer implant technology has improved refractive outcomes. For example, the <u>Toric lens</u> can now fix <u>astigmatism</u> and the <u>Restor lens</u> has a <u>fresnel lens</u> bifocal, which can help with near vision and decrease the need for <u>reading glasses</u>.

injections.
Several medicines are best delivered to the eye by injecting them directly into the <u>vitreous</u> cavity. The most common are the <u>anti-VEGF</u> medications like <u>Avastin</u> and <u>Lucentis</u> used for treating <u>macular degeneration</u>. <u>Steroids</u> such as <u>Kenalog</u> can also be injected into the eye for severe cases of <u>uveitis</u> and for decreasing inflammatory <u>macular edema</u>. Finally, with cases of internal eye infection (<u>endophthalmitis</u>), powerful <u>antibiotics</u> like <u>vancomycin</u> are typically injected directly into the eye to better target any infections.

Intralase.
This is an advance in LASIK surgery where the corneal flap is created using a <u>laser</u>. The older method of flap creation was using a microkeratome blade. Laser flap construction may decrease the chance of human errors in flap construction and makes LASIK surgery slightly safer. See <u>LASIK</u> and <u>femtosecond laser</u> for more information about this surgery.

intraocular pressure.
Also known as "IOP," this is the pressure inside the eye. We call this intraocular pressure to differentiate it from other kinds of pressure such as BP (blood pressure) and ICP (intracranial pressure) inside the skull. Normal eye pressure is 10-21. High pressure can cause <u>glaucoma</u> damage to the eye. See the entry on <u>pressure</u> for more information on this topic.

intraocular lens (IOL).
Also called an "IOL," this is the plastic lens placed into the eye during a <u>cataract surgery</u>. See <u>implant</u> for more information.

IOL-Master.
This is a machine used prior to <u>cataract surgery</u> to help determine the implant to use during surgery. With cataract surgery, the

cloudy cataract lens inside the eye is removed and must be replaced by a new lens implant. These implants come in different prescriptions, just like glasses or contact lenses. To help determine the proper implant prescription, the IOL-Master measures the length of the eye and the curvature of the cornea. This technology has removed much of the operator error with implant calculations (these used to be done by hand and were thus prone to mathematical or transcription errors). The IOL-Master has some limitations with cloudy cataracts and can't always measure through dense opacities in the lens. If this machine is unable to obtain a good eye measurement, a different (more involved) technique called immersion ultrasound (A-scan) can be used to measure the length of the eye prior to surgery.

ION. An ischemic optic neuropathy is a damaging event that happens in the optic nerve behind the eye when the blood supply to the nerve is temporarily blocked or interrupted. Without nutrition the nerve tissue swells and becomes damaged. Sudden and severe vision darkening occurs, often affecting either the upper or lower half of the vision. IONs tend to occur in middle age. While it is impossible to predict who will have an ION, some people have a "disk at risk" ... this is tight nerve insertion in the back of the eye seen during an eye exam. Something about this anatomy puts certain people at higher risk for an ION. While not a perfect metaphor, you can imagine that people who wear tight watch bands around their wrist will have more nerve damage if their arm ever swells up. There is no treatment for an ION, other than ruling out more serious conditions like temporal arteritis. The vision loss may improve with time. A new ION will often prompt a workup to look for vasculopathic risk factors like hypertension and diabetes. If the history warrants, we may also start an embolic workup to make sure the heart is beating normally (arrhythmias can cause clot formation) and a carotid ultrasound (to look for cholesterol emboli).

iris. The iris is the "colored" muscle inside the eye that controls pupil size. Some people have brown irises and others have blue. The color of the eye is determined by the amount of pigment in the iris, with dark brown eyes having more pigment than lighter eyes. The iris has rings of muscle fiber that contract and changes the pupil shape in response to light entering the eye. When inflamed, a condition called iritis, the iris can cause pain and sensitivity to light (photophobia). The iris is thin, like a drumhead, and very mobile. If the iris bows forward, the trabecular meshwork (the drain of the eye) may become blocked, leading to angle closure and acute glaucoma. Floppy iris syndrome (usually caused by urinary medications like Flomax) can cause difficulties during cataract surgery. Pupil abnormalities can occur from nerve blockage to the iris muscle from many sources including Horner's syndrome, Adie's pupil, third nerve palsy, or pharmacologic dilation.

iris synechiae.

This is an oddly shaped pupil that forms after inflammation inside the eye. The iris is the flat muscle inside our eye that controls pupil size and gives our eyes "color." When the iris is inflamed, such as after trauma or uveitis, it tends to become "sticky" and wants to scar to nearby structures. The pupil overlies the lens itself and if the edge of the pupil adheres to the lens underneath, the pupil will look abnormal. This adhesion is called a synechiae, and makes the pupil look like a cat's eye or a keyhole. If the adhesions are bad enough, the pupil can scar and create an acute glaucoma. In cases of ocular inflammation, we typically treat the eye with steroids to cool the eye down as quickly as possible. In addition, we may prescribe dilating drops to force the pupil to dilate and keep these adhesions from forming.

iritis.

This is inflammation of the iris, the "colored" part of the eye. The iris is a muscle that controls the size of the pupil. When inflamed, the iris muscle can "spasm" and cause intense eye pain. Most people with an iritis complain of extreme sensitivity to light (photophobia). Iris inflammation can occur from many sources such as trauma or after intraocular surgery. Another cause is uveitis. Uveitis is a similar (but more encompassing) term used to describe internal ocular inflammation, usually from pro-inflammatory systemic problems like sarcoidosis, rheumatoid arthritis, inflammatory bowel disease, and infection. Treatment for iritis involves topical steroids to "cool" the eye down. Cycloplegia dilating drops can help with iris pain by "paralyzing" the iris muscle so that it stops "spasming." Dilation drops are also helpful because they keep the pupil dilated and help avoid the formation of iris synechiae (this is when the iris inflammation causes it to 'stick' to nearby structures like the lens underneath).

ischemic optic neuropathy. This is damage to the <u>optic nerve</u> behind the eye that can occur in middle age. See <u>ION</u> for more information on this topic.

Istalol. This is the trade name for the <u>glaucoma</u> eye drop <u>timolol</u>. Timolol is a beta-blocker similar to the beta-blocker medicine used to control blood pressure. As this medicine has been around for a long time, it is also available as an inexpensive generic. Istalol comes in a thicker consistency, so the medicine lasts longer and is usually dosed once a day (as opposed to the twice a day dosing of the generic equivalent).

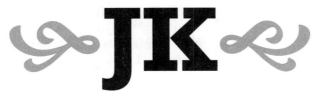

EYE CARTOON

by Tim Root, M.D.

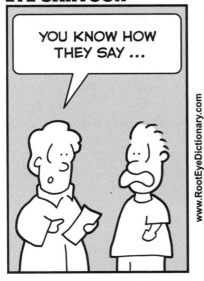

YOU KNOW HOW THEY SAY ...

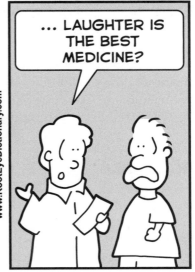

... LAUGHTER IS THE BEST MEDICINE?

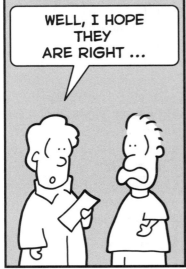

WELL, I HOPE THEY ARE RIGHT ...

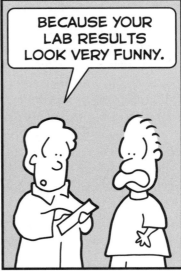

BECAUSE YOUR LAB RESULTS LOOK VERY FUNNY.

www.RootEyeDictionary.com

Copyright 2013 Root Eye Network, Inc.

Keflex. This is an oral <u>antibiotic</u> that is good for skin and sinus infections. Also known as <u>cephalexin</u>, it is relatively inexpensive and fairly effective. This medication is on the $4 list at Walmart and free at Publix supermarket.

Kenalog. This is a <u>steroid</u> that is used to decrease inflammation in the eye. Unlike other steroids we use in ophthalmology, this drug is delivered as an <u>injection</u>. We occasionally inject Kenalog into <u>chalazion</u> eyelid lesions to speed their resolution. For patients with resistant ocular inflammation (<u>uveitis</u>), Kenalog can be injected in the skin next to the eye or even behind the eye for continuous release. With <u>macular edema</u>, Kenalog is injected directly into the <u>vitreous</u> of the eye itself.

keratitis sicca. This is a fancy and erudite way of saying <u>dry eye</u>. Only pompous academics use this term.

keratoconus. This is an abnormal curvature of the <u>cornea</u> (the clear window that makes up the front of the eye). Normally, the cornea is spherical with a surface shape like a basketball. People with <u>astigmatism</u> have a cornea that is shaped like an American football. These shapes are easy to "fix" with <u>glasses</u>. Keratoconus is a whole different game. With this condition, the cornea weakens over time and takes on an irregular shape ... like that of a "beer belly" or a "pointy cone." This irregular surface creates optical aberrations that are impossible to correct using glasses. Hard <u>contacts</u> can be helpful, as they create a rounder 'surface' on the eye, but are difficult to fit. If bad enough, keratoconus eyes may require a <u>corneal transplant</u> to regain useful vision. The cause of keratoconus is believed to be from a defect in the collagen tissue that makes up the eye. Diagnosis is usually made with microscopic examination of the eye and by <u>corneal topography</u> (a machine that maps out the surface shape of the eye like a topographical map). People with keratoconus are poor candidates for <u>LASIK</u> as the laser procedure makes the cornea thinner and further weakens it.

keratometry. This is the technique used to measure the steepness of the cornea (the clear window that makes up the front of the eye.) Everyone has a different corneal steepness, and this variation has a large effect on the eye's overall focusing prescription. Normally, the cornea is perfectly round like the surface of a basketball. With astigmatism, however, the corneal surface is more like a football, and steeper along one axis while flatter along the other. Keratometry can measure this astigmatism. Keratometry measurements are important when fitting for contact lenses as contacts come with different "steepnesses" and they need to fit properly. Keratometry readings are also needed before cataract surgery in order to calculate the intraocular lens implants to use. Keratometry measurements can be performed manually or via automated machines (for example, the IOL-master machine used before cataract surgery).

ketotifen. This is a second generation antihistamine medication found in several of the better over-the-counter allergy eye drops. This medicine can be found at the store under the trade names Zaditor and Alaway. There are generic drops as well ... but not much cheaper than the brand names. Allergy medications like this are good for treating itchy eyes and ocular swelling. The half-life is about 12 hours, so this drop is commonly dosed twice a day.

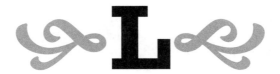

EYE CARTOON — by Tim Root, M.D.

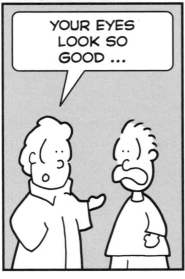

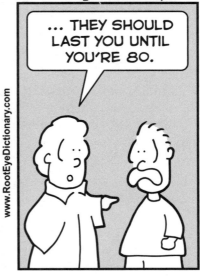

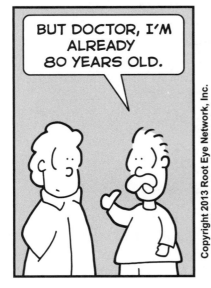

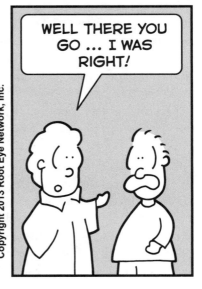

www.RootEyeDictionary.com

Copyright 2013 Root Eye Network, Inc.

lacrimal gland. The lacrimal gland is a tear-producing gland that is located in the upper eyelid, underneath the orbital bony ridge (i.e., under the bone that makes the upper eye socket). Most people think that the lacrimal gland is the main source of tears. Actually, that's not quite true. Most of the tears that cover our eyes are made by small accessory glands that cover the entire conjunctiva (the skin over the white of the eye) and under the eyelids. These little glands continuously excrete tears and create our "basal tear rate." The lacrimal gland is mostly responsible for reflexive tearing ... the tears that come out when crying or when the eyes are irritated. Many people with chronically dry eye complain that their eyes seem to water all the time. For these people, their basal tear rate is low so their eyes dry out and "sting" a little bit. This stinging causes the lacrimal gland to reflexively dump out all its tears at once, leading to episodes of excessive watering followed by periods of relative dryness. By breaking this dry-wet cycle with regular use of artificial tears, the lacrimal gland can calm down and decrease these unnecessary tearing episodes.

laser. Laser stands for "Light Amplification by Stimulated Emission of Radiation" (in case you were interested). Lasers work by amplifying light (or non-visible radiation) of a single wavelength. This can create a highly controllable beam of energy which can be used to burn, cut, or ablate tissues in the body. There are many uses for lasers in ophthalmology. The most obvious one is LASIK surgery, where a laser can be used to sculpt the surface of the cornea and fix a person's glasses prescription. Lasers are also used for treating after-cataracts, an opacity that can form after cataract surgery. The retina can be treated with a laser, and microaneurysms and edema from diabetic retinopathy can also be treated with a laser to stop the leakage (see FLT laser for more details). Retinal detachments can be "tacked down" with laser spots to keep the retina from peeling off further.

LASIK. This is a procedure where the cornea is sculpted with a laser in order to fix refractive error and decrease reliance on glasses. The cornea is the clear window that makes up the front of your eye. Surprisingly, the corneal surface does the majority of the light-focusing of the eye (not the lens inside the eye like you might expect). People with flat corneas have "weaker" powered eyes (hyperopia or farsightedness) while people with steep corneas have "over-powered" eyes (myopia or nearsightedness).

With LASIK, a special excimer laser is used to obliterate tissue and sculpt the cornea into the correct steepness. To minimize pain and inflammation, the laser is not applied directly to the surface of the eye. Instead, a partial thickness cut is made in the cornea to create a "flap." This flap is opened like a trapdoor to expose deeper layers of the corneal stroma underneath. The laser is then applied to this area to remove corneal tissue. When done, the corneal flap is flipped back over and "squeegeed" back into place to heal. While this may seem unnecessarily complicated, this flap method decreases inflammation and speeds healing time because the surface corneal epithelium is relatively intact. Because the treatment area is deep in the corneal tissue, it is more protected from problems (like scarring) while healing. There have been some more recent advances in the LASIK procedure ... one is Intralase where a femtosecond laser is used to create the flap (instead of the original microkeratome blade of the past). Not everyone is a good candidate for LASIK, such as those with keratoconus or naturally thin corneas (as measured by pachymetry). PRK is a similar to LASIK, but the laser is applied directly to the surface of the eye and thus has more post-operative discomfort and more potential for corneal haze (scaring).

Lastacaft. A prescription strength allergy drop good for treating swelling and itchy eyes. It is supposed to last about 16 hours, so is usually dosed once a day. Alternative prescription allergy drops include Bepreve and Pataday.

latanoprost. This is a prostaglandin eye drop used for treating glaucoma. The trade name is Xalatan. For many doctors, latanoprost is the first-line drop used in glaucoma because of its powerful effect and easy once-a-day dosing.

Latisse. This is a topical medicine used to make the eyelashes grow longer. This drug is the same medicine used in the glaucoma drop Lumigan (bimatoprost). Eyelash growth is a known side effect of prostaglandin glaucoma drops and Allergan is capitalizing on this with their topical product. Latisse is typically applied to the upper eyelid at night. While effective, especially compared to the "holistic" eyelash treatments on the market, there are some real side effects with this medicine you need to be aware of. First, the medicine can increase the pigmentation of the skin around the eyes, especially with long-term use. Another is that prostaglandins can cause a certain amount of redness and irritation to the eye itself - this is why it is applied at night so that you can sleep through any irritation. Also, this medicine can darken the eye color (the iris color) especially in people with hazel-colored eyes. Admittedly, we don't see these complications often in our practice, despite a large number of our patients on glaucoma drops. For our glaucoma patients the potential side effects are easy to justify - as glaucoma can cause blindness if not well-treated.

lattice degeneration. This is a thinning of the peripheral retina commonly found during a dilated eye exam. People with thinning retinas are at slightly higher risk for developing a retinal detachment in their lifetime. This localized area of atrophy is predisposed to forming holes or tears (especially after a vitreous detachment) that can extend into the rest of the eye. Lattice degeneration is very common with about 5% of the population demonstrating this finding, especially in people with large amounts of nearsightedness.

lazy eye. This is an eye that doesn't see well but is otherwise healthy. This occurs from disuse at a young age when the visual nervous system is still forming. See amblyopia for more information on this topic.

legal blindness. In North America, the definition of legal blindness is vision that is 20/200 or less in the best seeing eye, despite using the best correction possible (i.e., up-to-date glasses). A 20/200 vision measurement on the Snellen chart means that if a "legally blind person" stood 20 feet away from a vision chart, they could read only as good as a "normal person" standing 200 feet away. Another definition of legal blindness is used for people with severely constricted peripheral vision (typically 20 degrees or less). These people may have good central vision on an eye chart, but their peripheral vision is so constricted that its like they are looking through a "soda straw." This amount of vision is unsafe for driving (or duck hunting) so it is *also* called "legal blindness."

lens. The lens is the magnifying glass inside our eye that controls fine focusing. The lens is located immediately behind the <u>iris</u> (the colored part of the eye). Like the <u>cornea</u>, it is living tissue yet it is clear. When light enters the eye, it travels through the pupil, then through the lens, before striking the <u>retina</u> in the back of the eye. The lens is held in place by little springs called <u>zonules</u>. These are arranged in a 360-degree ring around the lens "equator" and suspend the lens like a trampoline. A muscle called the <u>ciliary body</u> pulls on the zonules which controls the lens shape. This shape-changing ability is called <u>accommodation</u>, which is how we focus to see things close up. In youth, the lens is naturally soft and can change shape like a piece of Jell-O or gummy candy. This gives children a very wide range of focus as their lens can flatten like a 'pancake' to give far distance vision, or the lens can become round like a 'marble' to focus on the tip of a nose. As we age, the clear lens tissue begins to stiffen, and has a harder time changing shape. This process is called <u>presbyopia</u>, and explains why we start needing reading glasses around age 40. The lens eventually becomes cloudy, forming a <u>cataract</u>. When we repair a cataract, we create a hole in the front layer of the lens and remove the inner layers of the lens. A new plastic <u>implant</u> lens is then placed inside the husk of the original cataract lens. This new implant is optically clear, but made of plastic that can't change shape, so most are therefore set for one focus (to give good distance vision).

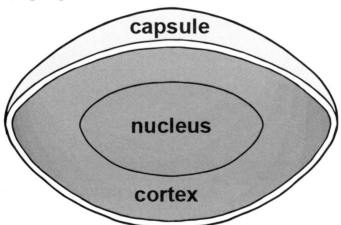

The lens has three layers. Cataract opacities often
form in the inner nucleus layer.

105

lensometer. A machine used in an eye doctor's office that can measure the prescription in an existing pair of glasses. Some are manual and others are automated machines. Knowing your current glasses prescription gives us a starting point when performing refraction (checking your vision on the eye chart). This measurement also allows us to advise you whether it's worth it to update your spectacles ... after all, if your new prescription is the same as your existing glasses, you might not want to bother purchasing another pair.

levobunolol. A glaucoma eye drop. This is a beta-blocker similar to the eye drop timolol. This drop is generic and inexpensive, but I don't use it often as timolol is readily available.

lidocaine. This is an anesthetic liquid that is commonly injected into the skin prior to surgical procedures. I use it most commonly with chalazion excisions or when removing a papilloma from the eyelid. We inject lidocaine inside the eye during cataract surgery to numb the iris. On occasion, I will inject the medication behind the eye when performing a retrobulbar block - these blocks are only performed prior to difficult cataract surgeries, however.

lid scrubs. This is a technique for cleaning the eyelids in order to improve comfort, especially in cases of blepharitis. Debris can form on the eyelashes. This debris is typically made of dead skin cells and dried-up tear secretions. It is harmless, but bacteria living on our skin like to eat this debris because it is like "free lunch" to them. These bacteria create their own waste products that irritate the skin of the eyelids, making them puffy, red, and giving the eyes a sandy sensation. This is called blepharitis and is very common. If we improve our lid "hygiene" and remove some of this debris, the eyes will feel better and less irritated. There are many ways to accomplish this. You can take a soft washcloth, dip it in warm water and add a little baby shampoo, and use this to gently scrub the lash line (with the eyes closed of course). You can also make a mixture of diluted baby shampoo and do the same regimen with cotton balls. Finally, there are pre-made pads such as the OCuSOFT pads, that are already prepared and ready for use. I usually recommend doing this lid scrub only once a day (though some people prefer more often). If you wash your lashes *too* often you may reach a point where your scrubbing regimen is irritating the lids more than it is actually helping.

Lotemax. This is the trade name for the steroid loteprednol. This steroid eye drop is commonly used after cataract surgery and in cases of ocular inflammation. While not quite as strong as prednisolone, Lotemax is touted as a safer medicine as it has less steroid side effects like increased eye pressure.

loteprednol. A popular steroid eye drop that is usually packaged under the trade name Lotemax. This drop is commonly used in cases of ocular inflammation and for use after eye surgery to cool the eye down. This drug is also available in lower concentrations in the drop Alrex.

low-tension glaucoma. This is glaucoma that occurs despite the eye pressure being "normal." Glaucoma is normally defined as high intraocular pressure that causes damage to the optic nerve over many years. The underlying mechanism behind glaucoma is poorly understood but high pressure seems to be the main instigator. Some people seem to be exquisitely sensitive to mild pressure and develop nerve damage despite their eye pressure being in the "normal" range (10 to 21). These people require treatment to keep pressures very low. This is done with eye drops, lasers, and rarely glaucoma surgery.

LPI. This is the abbreviation for Laser Peripheral Iridotomy, a laser procedure performed on people who are at risk for having an acute glaucoma attack. To understand the purpose behind this procedure, it can be useful to think of the eye like a kitchen sink full of water. There is a "faucet" running at all times inside the eye that produces aqueous fluid. This fluid keeps the eye inflated like a water balloon and working properly. There is also a "drain" in the eye called the trabecular meshwork where the aqueous fluid drains away. It is the balance of this fluid input and output that determines the eye's pressure. The eye's drain is located in a 360-degree ring at the intersection of the iris (colored part of the eye) with the sclera (the white part of the eye). This intersection is commonly called the "angle" because it is a rather tight intersection with little excess room. Some people's ocular anatomy is such that their drainage angle is extremely tight and narrow. Under most situations, aqueous fluid can still drain out this tight junction ... but if conditions are just right, the drainage angle may shut closed entirely. With the drainage pathway blocked, the eye pressure will shoot up and cause intense pain with vision loss from acute glaucoma. This is always a bad situation ... most people come into the office bent over and throwing up from the pain. Even with prompt treatment there is usually some permanent vision loss. For people who appear to have <u>narrow angles</u>, a prophylactic LPI is sometimes recommended. With this procedure a laser is used to create a small hole through the iris. This helps equalize the pressures inside the eye and dramatically decreases the chance of having an acute glaucoma episode. The laser procedure is quick, and for the most part harmless, though there are a couple of risks to be aware of. The main one is visual side effects afterwards. By creating a hole in the iris, this creates a secondary <u>pupil</u> that light can pass through to reach the retina. Some people complain of a ghost image or line around lights at night. This is rare, and we strive to keep the LPI hole very small and up under the eyelid to minimize this possibility. This must be considered and weighed against the possibility of a potentially blinding glaucoma attack.

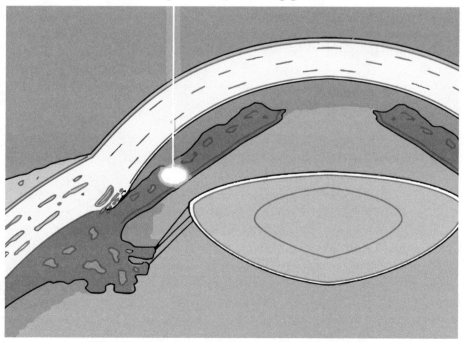

With LPI, a laser creates a hole through the iris to avoid the possibility of angle-closure glaucoma.

Lucentis. This is an injectable anti-VEGF medicine used primarily to treat wet macular degeneration. It works by decreasing fluid release from leaking blood vessels under the retina. Lucentis is touted as being a more selective medicine than its competitor Avastin (and Lucentis costs a premium for this reason).

Lumigan. A prostaglandin eye drop used for treating glaucoma. The active ingredient is bimatoprost. Like all the prostaglandins, this medicine is dosed only once a day and usually taken in the evening. Similar medications include Xalatan (latanoprost) and Travatan (travoprost).

lutein. This is a yellow pigment created by plants that is absorbed and used by animals. Lutein is found in animal fats and is what gives egg yolks that yellow color. It is found in the retina along with another similar pigment called zeaxanthin. Lutein and zeaxanthin supplementation has been studied and found to be beneficial with macular degeneration (see the AREDS 2 Study for more information on this topic).

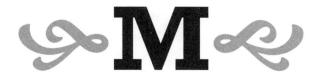

EYE CARTOON
by Tim Root, M.D.

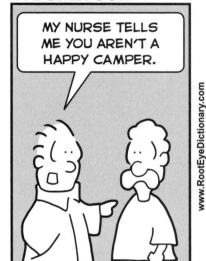

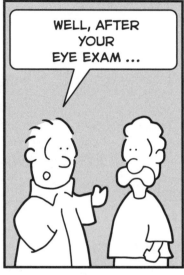

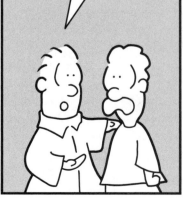

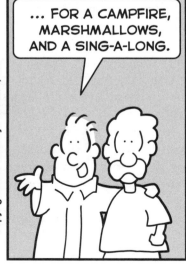

www.RootEyeDictionary.com

Copyright 2013 Root Eye Network, Inc.

Macugen. An anti-VEGF injection medicine used in the treatment of wet macular degeneration. This medicine is being supplanted by other drugs in the same class such as Avastin (cheaper) and Lucentis/Eylea (possibly more effective).

macula. The macula is the part of the retina that is responsible for our fine central vision. This is the vision necessary for reading a book, watching television, or seeing distant road signs. The retina works like film in a camera, and the macula is the most sensitive part of the film, containing more rod and cone photoreceptors than elsewhere. Problems at the macula, such as diabetic retinopathy or macular degeneration, can cause severe visual changes (though the peripheral vision remains intact). The macula can be viewed through dilation. The macula can also be measured using OCT photographs to look for swelling or sub-retinal bleeding. When there are problems, such as wet macular degeneration, the circulation under and around the macula can be further imaged using fluorescein angiogram (though this type of testing is usually left to retinal specialists).

macular degeneration. Macular degeneration is premature aging of the retina. The retina is located in the back of the eye and works like "the film in a camera," detecting light and images. The macula is the central retina responsible for fine central vision. If the macular retina wears down this can cause serious problems. For most people, this results in difficulty seeing fine details such as small type in books ... though ARMD can cause serious vision loss when advanced. Most people have dry macular degeneration where the vision slowly worsens with time. Treatment for dry degeneration is limited, and revolves around using eye vitamins and vision screening with an Amsler grid at home and OCT scans at our office. Some people go on to develop wet macular degeneration where the retinal blood vessels leak fluid and this can lead to rapid vision loss. Wet degeneration causes significant vision changes, but there are also more treatment options such as anti-VEGF injections and laser. Wet degeneration can be detected with OCT scans and leaky areas further localized using fluorescein angiography.

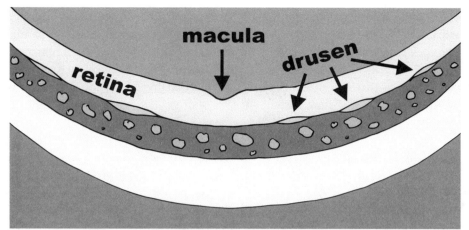

"Dry" macular degeneration involves the formation of drusen under the retina that lead to gradual retinal atrophy and vision loss over time.

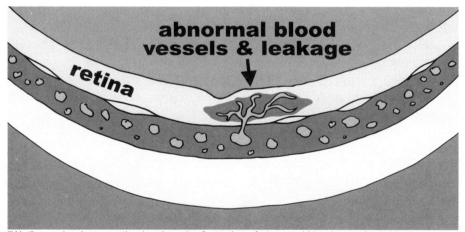

"Wet" macular degeneration involves the formation of abnormal blood vessels and leakage within the retina. This leads to sudden and rapid vision loss.

macular edema. This is swelling of the <u>macula</u>, the area of the <u>retina</u> that is responsible for our fine central vision. The retina can be thought of like film in a camera. Just like film, the retina needs to be perfectly smooth and flat if we are going to "take a good picture" and see clearly. If there is swelling at the macula, then the "film" becomes distorted in the middle and this creates blur or distortion to the central vision as well. There are many causes of macular edema, such as leaking vessels from <u>wet macular degeneration</u>, <u>diabetic retinopathy</u>, or traction from <u>epiretinal membranes</u>. Retinal edema can be detected in our office using <u>OCT</u> photographs to map out the retinal surface. Early retinal changes may even be detected at home using an <u>Amsler grid</u>. Treatment for this condition depends upon the cause, but usually involves <u>injections</u> of anti-inflammatory medications (such as <u>Kenalog</u> or <u>Avastin</u>) if there is active bleeding or if the edema is not resolving.

macular hole. This is a small hole that forms in the <u>macula</u> that creates significant vision problems. The <u>retina</u> is located in the back of the eye and acts like film in a camera. The macula is the most important part of the retina as it is responsible for our fine central vision. If a hole forms in this area, the central vision "goes to pot." There are several causes for a macular hole. One is an <u>epiretinal membrane</u>. This is a clear fibrous membrane that can form on the surface of the retina with age (and sometimes after trauma). This membrane can contract like "shrink-wrap plastic" and cause traction on the retinal surface. This creates wrinkles on the surface of the retina and if bad enough, can pull open a full-thickness hole in the macula. A hole can also form from the traction of a <u>vitreous detachment</u>. The <u>vitreous</u> is the gel that fills the rear chamber of the eye. The vitreous has a tendency to contract and collapse inwards with age, tugging on the retina. This can create retinal tears or holes and lead to a <u>retinal detachment</u>. If this tugging occurs at the macula, a full thickness hole can result. Macular holes, if small enough, may close on their own but often require surgical correction. This usually involves a <u>membrane peel</u> surgery. In this surgery, a <u>retina specialist</u> will enter through the back of the eye and remove the source of the traction (i.e., remove the epiretinal membrane or vitreous jelly). Then, a gas bubble is injected into the eye in order to smooth out the retina, and (hopefully) the hole will close over the next several weeks. Though a commonly performed surgery, membrane peels are not always successful. A macular hole causes central vision distortion that can be detected with an <u>OCT</u> scan of the retina. <u>Amsler grid</u> monitoring at home may pick up an early macular hole as well, but definitive diagnosis is made in the doctor's office.

macular pucker. This is a membrane that forms on the surface of the <u>retina</u> that causes it to wrinkle or "pucker." Other names for this are epiretinal membrane and cellophane retinopathy. See the entry on epiretinal membrane for a more detailed explanation of this common finding.

Malyugin ring. This is a small spring-like device used during cataract surgery to help dilate the pupil. Small pupils make cataract surgery difficult, as the procedure involves vacuuming out the cataract "through" the pupil. Some people have naturally small pupils (the black hole in the middle of the iris) and don't dilate well. Poor dilation may be genetic or occur from atrophy of the iris muscle that occurs with age. The smaller the pupil, the more difficult it is to work on the cataract. In these cases, many surgeons will use a Malyugin ring. It is a small spring made of plastic that is temporarily injected into the eye to keep the pupil wide open (with a mild amount of iris stretching) until the surgery is completed. At the end of the surgery, the ring is removed to allow the pupil to constrict back to its normal size. This is a simple yet elegant technique that is also useful in cases of floppy iris syndrome as the ring keeps the iris from moving around during surgery.

Maxitrol. This is a combination of neomycin/polymyxin (antibiotics) and dexamethasone (a mild steroid). This antibiotic combination comes in both drop and ointment forms and is useful for mild infection or inflammation such as blepharitis. Some people are sensitive to the neomycin and may require more expensive alternative drugs like Tobradex or Zylet. Maxitrol is generic and on the $4 generic list at Walmart.

meibomian glands. These are small glands that run along the edge of the upper and lower eyelid. Meibomian glands produce oil that is continuously excreted into the tear film. This oil keeps the tears slippery and also forms a protective "evaporation proof" barrier on the surface of the tear film. The meibomian gland pore openings are small, and can't easily be seen without a microscope. If a meibomian gland pore gets clogged, the oil can back up into the eyelid and form a chalazion. Chalazions will sometimes spontaneously drain with the use of warm compresses and massage but will sometimes require surgical drainage in the office. Blepharitis is a condition where chronic eyelid irritation makes the eyes look puffy and feel sandy. Blepharitis also tends to clog the

meibomian glands, which is why warm compresses and massage are often recommended for this condition as well ... to keep the meibomian glands flowing properly.

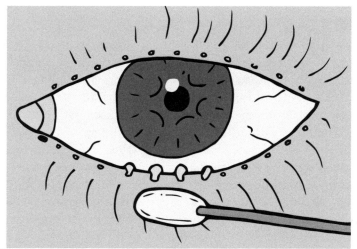

Meibomian glands produce oil that is continuously injected into the tear film.

membrane peel. This is a surgery performed by a <u>retinal specialist</u> to remove an epiretinal membrane from the eye. An <u>epiretinal membrane</u> is a clear membrane that can form on the <u>retina</u>. While normally innocuous, this membrane may contract and can make the retinal surface "wrinkled" leading to vision loss. With a membrane peel surgery, the retina doctor goes into the eye and gently peels this membrane off to relieve traction. Then, a gas bubble is typically injected into the eye. This gas bubble lasts for several weeks and is designed to gently press on the retina and flatten the retina back into a smooth configuration. Since gas floats, a patient may be required to keep their head in a downward position for several weeks. This positioning can be a little harsh on the body, and patients come back to our office looking a little disheveled. This inconvenience is worth it if some vision is regained. Membrane peel surgery is not always successful, so most retina doctors like to wait until the vision deteriorates to a point they feel that the "benefits outweigh the risks" for the operation.

metal foreign body. This is a piece of metal in the eye, and is commonly caused while grinding or working on machinery. Small pieces of metal can fly or fall into the eye, and for some reason, metal likes to stick to the clear <u>cornea</u>. When this happens, the metal will embed into the eye and rust into place (the <u>tear film</u> is rather salty). Metal in the eye is painful and if not removed promptly, can lead to infection and scarring with potential long-term visual consequences. Sometimes, a piece of metal can be wiped off with a cotton swab, but often it requires more aggressive debridement. Typically, we'll numb the eye with topical <u>anesthesia drops</u>. Then, a small metal pick (like a needle, but not sharp) is used to wipe the piece off the cornea. If there is residual rust or metal fragments, this may need to be removed with a high-speed rotary tool like a microscopic dremel tool. This is all done sitting up at the exam chair, and while most people are understandably nervous, the whole procedure is surprisingly pain-free. Afterwards, we treat with <u>antibiotics</u> and recheck the eye over the next week to make sure no infection occurs. If, based on history and exam findings, we are concerned about a piece of metal actually penetrating the eye ... then a more involved examination is done. This may require a CAT scan to rule out metal pieces inside the eyeball.

methazolamide. Also known by the trade name <u>Neptazane</u>, this is a water pill used in the treatment of <u>glaucoma</u>. It is a <u>carbonic anhydrase inhibitor</u> that works by decreasing the production of <u>aqueous</u> fluid inside the eye. This medicine has the same mechanism of action of <u>Diamox</u> (acetazolamide).

migraine aura. This is a visual distortion that can occur during or before a migraine headache. Migraines are bad headaches associated with sensitivity to light or sound (and often nausea). Like most headaches, the underlying mechanism is not entirely understood but migraines may occur because of spasm of blood vessels in the brain. With some people, the spasming vessels occur at the back of the brain near the occipital cortex. This is the part of the brain that processes our vision, and when irritated, the occipital cortex can create visual hallucinations. Most people describe an "aura" to their vision where the center of their vision (or perhaps more to the side) becomes blurry. They may see lights, sparkles, or geometric distortions like a kaleidoscope. These visual changes tend to expand and spread to one side before subsiding after 15 to 30 minutes. Afterwards, some people get the traditional migraine headache, but other people have the visual symptoms alone with no

residual discomfort. Migraine auras can be scary but are rarely serious. Some people are worried when their visual symptoms "change sides" and occur on the other half of the vision. This is actually a good sign, however, as variation is typical for migraines. It's when you have the *same* visual phenomenon over and over, always in the same place that we have to consider other possibilities like a mass lesion that is tickling the occipital lobe in one spot. In these cases, an MRI is obtained.

monocular precautions. Many people have only one good eye. Despite this limitation, they live perfectly rich and normal lives. We recommend these fine people take extra precautionary steps to keep their good eye "healthy." For example, if a rock randomly strikes you in the eye you don't have a backup eye to rely on. Conversely, if you get in a car accident, it would be nice to have some additional protection from flying glass. Monocular precautions usually involves safety <u>glasses</u> or getting your prescription glasses made of polycarbonate plastic (which acts like safety glass). If you wear <u>contacts</u>, then good hygiene becomes especially important as you don't want to get an infection in your only eye.

monovision. With monovision, one eye is set for distance vision while the other is set for near. Many <u>contact</u> lens wearers use a "monovision contact prescription" to avoid <u>reading glasses</u>. Most will set their dominant eye for distance and their non-dominant eye set for reading. While some people tolerate this imbalance well, other people hate monovision. The disparity between their eyes makes them sick to their stomach and unsteady on their feet. The blur at distance ruins their depth perception for driving, and reading becomes a chore because one eye is doing all the work. With <u>LASIK</u> or <u>cataract surgery</u> we have the opportunity to change your eyes' prescription. Some people choose to have monovision after surgery as they have tolerated it well in the past.

Moxeza. This is the trade name for the antibiotic <u>moxifloxacin</u>. This is a powerful <u>antibiotic</u> eye drop commonly used after <u>cataract surgery</u> and for more serious eye infections (such as a <u>corneal ulcer</u> in a contact lens wearer).

moxifloxacin. This is a powerful fluoroquinolone antibiotic eye drop, commonly used after cataract surgery and more serious eye infections (especially in contact lens wearers). This antibiotic is available under the trade names Vigamox and Moxeza.

MRI. MRI stands for magnetic resonance imaging. An MRI uses a large magnet and radio fields to view the interior body. MRI is particularly good at imaging soft tissues like the brain, but has limited use for looking at the eye itself. Some scientists estimate that a third of the brain is involved with vision in some way. Therefore, we obtain an MRI in cases of unexplained visual field loss or with cranial nerve palsies to look for tumors, mass lesions, and signs of stroke.

multifocal contact. This is a contact lens that is designed to improve both distance and near vision. The contact has separate zones of focus to accomplish this, arranged in a concentric ring like a fresnel lens. The downside to multifocal contacts is that they may not work perfectly for everyone and they are not quite as clear as a regular contact or glasses. The alternative is monovision, with one eye set for distance and the other set for near.

multifocal implant. This is an implant used during cataract surgery that may eliminate the need for reading glasses. With cataract surgery, the cloudy lens inside the eye is removed and replaced with a plastic implanted lens. The standard implant most people choose is focused for distance vision. These people continue to need bifocals or reading glasses after surgery for near vision. New "premium" implants are now available that have a bifocal built into them. There are different zones built into the implant surface that focus at different distances. These "multifocal implants" have more out-of-pocket expense than a standard lens because insurance companies will not pay for the additional cost. Not everyone is a good candidate for this type of lens as there are some small tradeoffs with multifocal implants. They may not be as crisp as a traditional lens and many people see ring-halos at night. Currently, the leading multifocal implant on the market is the Restor lens. A competing product called the Crystalens gives a similar focal effect, but works by a completely different mechanism. Most surgeons have a preference on the type of implant they use.

multiple sclerosis. An inflammatory disorder of the nervous system characterized by multiple neurologic symptoms over time. Multiple sclerosis (MS) occurs because of inflammation of the nerves in the body and brain. A myelin sheath normally surrounds the nerves in the body, acting just like the "insulation" on electrical wires. With MS, inflammation causes this insulation to break down, effectively "short circuiting" the normal nerve transmission. The eye is one of the areas most often affected as the optic nerve contains over a million individual nerve fibers. Inflammation in this nerve causes vision problems - this is called optic neuritis and is often one of the first symptoms of MS.

Muro 128. This is a hyperosmotic (lots of salt) eye drop that is used in cases of corneal edema. The cornea (the clear structure that makes up the front of our eye) is clear because it is relatively dry. With certain conditions such as Fuchs' dystrophy or after cataract surgery, the cornea can become wet and cloudy. Muro drops and ointments can be used to dry the eye out. Because this drop has a high salt content, water is attracted to it and the drop literally sucks or pulls water out of the cornea. Muro isn't really a drug so you don't necessarily need a prescription for it. However, pharmacists keep it behind the counter and so a prescription is usually written anyway.

myasthenia gravis. This is a rare autoimmune disease that causes easy fatigue of muscles throughout the body. When muscle fatigue occurs in the eye, this creates intermittent double vision (diplopia) and droopy eyelids (ptosis), especially when tired later in the day. The mechanism of this disorder involves the body developing antibodies to its own muscle nerve receptors. The eye muscles seem to be especially susceptible to this fatigue and this disorder is often first diagnosed at the eye doctor's office. More definitive diagnosis is made by a neurologist who looks for certain blood markers and performs electrical muscle stimulation tests. Primary doctors are also involved to check thyroid levels and insure the thymus gland is healthy.

Mydriacyl. This is the trade name for the dilating drop tropicamide. This is a short-acting dilating drop used during an eye exam to dilate the pupil. This drop also has cycloplegia effects which means that it will cause a fair amount of blurriness (especially with reading). It is the shortest acting dilator available, but even so, the dilation/blur can last anywhere from 3-8 hours.

myopia. This is another way of saying an eye is nearsighted. See the entry of nearsightedness for more information.

N

EYE CARTOON

by Tim Root, M.D.

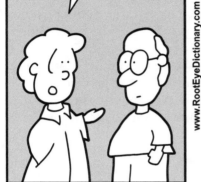

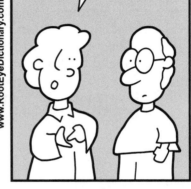

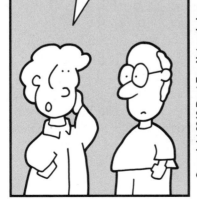

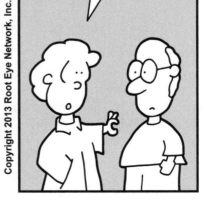

naphazoline. This is a vasoconstrictor found in many over-the-counter eye drops such as <u>Naphcon-A</u> and <u>Opcon-A</u>. By constricting the blood vessels on the <u>conjunctiva</u> surface, this makes the eyes look whiter. Unfortunately, many people develop a rebound redness and their eyes actually look more red and swollen when the drop wears off. We see a similar response with <u>Visine</u> ... which is why most eye doctors don't recommend using vasoconstrictors.

Naphcon-A. This is an over-the-counter <u>allergy drop</u>, useful for itching and swelling of the <u>eyelids</u>. This drop actually contains two separate drugs. The first is called <u>pheniramine</u> - this is an antihistamine to decrease inflammation. While effective, it is not as powerful as stronger antihistamines found in newer drops. The other drug is called <u>naphazoline</u>. This is a vasoconstrictor that makes the eyes less red, but can cause a rebound redness when the drop wears off (an effect similar to <u>Visine</u>). Overall, Naphcon-A and the other generic equivalents are effective but I never prescribe them as they are not as powerful as newer allergy drops like <u>Alaway</u>/<u>Zaditor</u> or the prescription drops <u>Bepreve</u> and <u>Pataday</u>.

narrow angles. This is when the "<u>angle</u>" inside the eye is naturally tight, putting you at risk for having an acute <u>glaucoma</u> attack. The front part of the eye is filled with a fluid called the <u>aqueous</u> humor. This fluid is continuously produced and drained from the eye, with the balance of fluid input and output controlling the overall <u>pressure</u> of the eye. The drain inside the eye is called the <u>trabecular meshwork</u> and it is located where the white of the eye (the <u>sclera</u>) meets the colored <u>iris</u>. The anatomy of this intersection forms an angle. Some people's ocular anatomy is such that their angle is very narrow. If the angle narrows too much, it can shut down entirely. With no aqueous drainage, the pressure inside the eye shoots up suddenly, causing an <u>acute glaucoma</u> with extreme pain and vision loss. Narrow angles can be evaluated using <u>gonioscopy</u>. If the angles are narrow enough, a prophylactic <u>LPI</u> procedure can be considered to avoid angle closure.

nasolacrimal duct obstruction. This is a blockage of the tear drainage pathway that connects the eye to the nose. Tears are produced in the eyelids and cover the eye like a waterfall. Because of gravity, tears eventually form a small "lake" running along the edge of the lower eyelid. This lake drains through little holes in the eyelid called puncta, through some "underground tubing" in the skin and eventually into the nose. This drainage pathway is called the nasolacrimal system, and is the reason when we have runny eyes, we tend to have a runny nose as well. If this pathway becomes blocked, the tears have nowhere to drain, instead welling up in the eye and even running down the cheek. In adults, nasolacrimal duct (NLD) obstruction can be temporary if from allergic soft tissue swelling or permanent if caused by scarring from a prior infection. Many children are born with a temporary NLD obstruction at birth that eventually resolves during the first year (but may also require probing to manually force open). In adults, NLD obstruction often requires a surgical procedure called a dacryocystorhinostomy (DCR for short). This surgery involves making a small incision on the skin and creating a new drainage pathway for the tears to enter the nose. This type of procedure is usually performed by an oculoplastic surgeon, though occasionally ENT doctors will perform the same procedure.

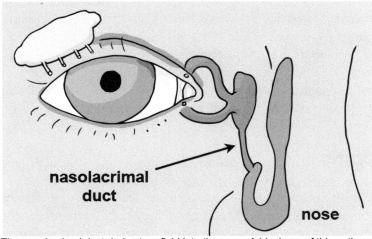

The nasolacrimal duct drains tear fluid into the nose. A blockage of this pathway may cause excessive tears that run down the cheek instead.

Natamycin. Also known as pimaricin, this is the only commercially prepared eye drop available for fungal eye infection. While effective, it can sometimes be hard to obtain and can be expensive. The main

alternative we use is <u>amphotericin B</u> ... but this drug isn't easy to obtain either as it has to be especially prepared by a compounding pharmacy.

nearsightedness. This is a refractive error where the eyes see well at near distance, but have a hard time seeing far away. Normally, the eye works like a camera with light entering the eye being focused perfectly on the <u>retina</u>. The retina is analogous to the film in a camera and located at the back of the eye. When a person is nearsighted, however, light wants to focus in front of the retina and visual images look blurry. By weakening the eye's overall focusing power with glasses (using negative <u>diopter</u> power lenses) light can focus properly on the retina. Extremely nearsighted eyes tend to be longer or larger than average, which puts them at slightly increased risk for <u>retinal detachment</u>. The prevalence of nearsightedness seems to be increasing in our society ... the reason for this is not entirely clear, but it may have something to do with the increase in near activities (i.e., iPads and Game Boys).

Neomycin/Polymyxin/Dexamethasone - An inexpensive combination drop containing two <u>antibiotics</u> to treat infection combined with a mild <u>steroid</u> for inflammation. This drug is available as an eye drop or an ointment. While most tolerate this medicine, some people have a sensitivity to the neomycin component. For these people, <u>Tobradex</u> or <u>Zylet</u> may be a better option. The trade name for this medicine is <u>Maxitrol</u>, which is still used to describe this medicine as it is easier to pronounce. This drug is on the $4 generic list at Walmart.

Neosporin. This is a combination <u>antibiotic</u> ointment containing neomycin, <u>bacitracin</u>, and <u>polymyxin</u>. While relatively effective as a broad spectrum antibiotic, some people have an allergy or sensitivity to neomycin. In these cases, <u>Polysporin</u> (which only contains bacitracin and polymyxin) can be used to good effect. I rarely prescribe this medicine given the plethora of good antibiotic drops and ointments available that have less side effects.

neovascularization. This is when abnormal blood vessels grow inside the eye. The eye is a very metabolically active organ. It continuously works and detects light, even while sleeping. In some ways

the eye works like the heart ... in the sense that it is "always on." As such, the eye, especially the retina, requires a rich blood supply to function properly. The retina doesn't have a collateral blood supply. It only gets its blood and oxygen nourishment from a couple of sources. If there is a disruption to this blood supply, the retina quickly becomes starved for oxygen and can die. Many things can disrupt the blood flow to the eye. Diabetic retinopathy, blood clots, and macular degeneration can interfere with the blood supply to the retina. In all of these cases, the retina becomes "hungry" for oxygen and responds by pumping out "vascular endothelial growth factors" or VEGFs. These are natural hormonal stimulants for the growth of new blood vessels inside the eye. Normally, this would be great as new blood vessels could bring in fresh blood and keep the retina well-nourished, but it doesn't work this way. The new blood vessels grow quickly and are abnormal, with a tendency to leak, bleed, and contract causing vitreous hemorrhages, macular edema, and even retinal detachments. It is the VEGFs that cause neovascularization. To combat neovascularization, eye doctors try to decrease VEGF production. PRP laser can be performed to destroy these tissues. For more localized neovascularization at the macula, anti-VEGF injection medicines like Avastin are now being used extensively in the eye and this has drastically improved the treatment for "wet" macular degeneration.

neovascular glaucoma.

With neovascularization, abnormal blood vessels grow inside the eye, causing significant retinal damage. These blood vessels can also grow into the front of the eye, covering the surface of the iris, and into the trabecular meshwork drain. If this drain becomes blocked with abnormal vessels, aqueous fluid can't exit back into the blood stream. This causes extremely high pressure inside, leading to acute glaucoma. Neovascular glaucoma is very difficult to treat as the pressure is recalcitrant to normal glaucoma drops. In these cases, a tube-shunt procedure is often required to create a new drainage pathway out of the eye. There are several causes for neovascular glaucoma but the most common is after a central retinal vein occlusion.

nepafenac.

Known by the trade name Nevanac, this is an anti-inflammatory NSAID eye drop that is commonly used after cataract surgery to cool the eye down and decrease the chance of macular edema.

Neptazane. Also called <u>methazolamide</u>, this is a water pill used in the treatment of <u>glaucoma</u>. It is a <u>carbonic anhydrase inhibitor</u> that works by decreasing the production of <u>aqueous</u> fluid inside the eye. This medicine has the same mechanism of action as <u>Diamox</u> (<u>acetazolamide</u>).

Nevanac. Also known as <u>nepafenac</u>, this is an <u>NSAID</u> anti-inflammatory eye drop. It is commonly used after <u>cataract surgery</u> to cool the eye down and decrease the risk of post-operative <u>macular edema</u>.

NSAID. This stands for Non-Steroidal Anti-Inflammatory Drug. NSAIDs are very common. In fact, most over the counter pain relievers such as aspirin, Motrin (ibuprofen), and Tylenol are NSAIDs. In the eye, NSAID eye drops are used for pain control, but are most often used after <u>cataract surgery</u> to decrease the possibility of <u>macular edema</u>. Common NSAID eye drops include <u>Acular</u>, <u>Nevanac</u>, <u>diclofenac</u>, and <u>Bromday</u>.

numbing drops. These are eye drops used to anesthetize the surface of the eye. They are commonly used during an eye exam to help check the eye <u>pressure</u> (see <u>applanation tonometry</u>) and to numb the eye prior to eye surgery. See <u>anesthetic drops</u> for more information on this topic.

nystagmus. This is an involuntary, rhythmic "to and fro" movement of the eyes. Most nystagmus are in the horizontal axis, such that the eyes are constantly moving to the left and right. There are many causes for this abnormal eye movement, though most nystagmus occur secondary to congenital motor deficits that begin in childhood. Sensory nystagmus can occur in a child who is born with poor vision and is associated with many other congenital visual defects such as albinism. Nystagmus that develop later in life are rare and can be caused by vestibular (inner ear) abnormalities, drug toxicities (including alcohol), or more serious neurologic problems like a tumor or stroke. Police officers sometimes look for nystagmus with their field sobriety tests, looking for horizontal nystagmus while asking people to look to their right and left.

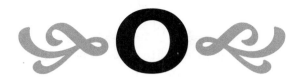

EYE CARTOON

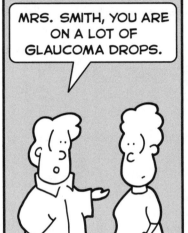

MRS. SMITH, YOU ARE ON A LOT OF GLAUCOMA DROPS.

TO HELP WITH COMPLIANCE, I'D LIKE TO CONSOLIDATE YOUR MEDICATIONS.

WE'VE MIXED ALL OF YOUR EYE DROPS INTO A SINGLE BOTTLE.

USE THIS TWICE A DAY. YOU MAY REQUIRE SOME ASSISTANCE.

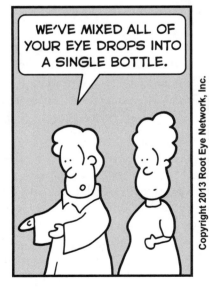
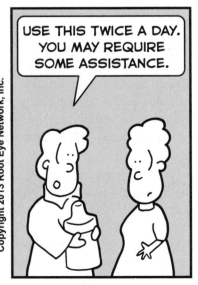

www.RootEyeDictionary.com

Copyright 2013 Root Eye Network, Inc.

OCT. Also known as Optical Coherence Tomography, this is a machine used to take a picture and "map" the surface contour of the retina. It works very similar to ultrasound, but instead of using sound, light waves are bounced off the internal eye structures. The scans produced by this machine look similar to that produced by a sonar depth finder in a boat ... but instead of mapping the bottom of the ocean or river bed, we are measuring the surface of the retina (which is supposed to be flat and smooth like film in a camera). OCT is useful for detecting retinal distortions (like those caused by an epiretinal membrane) and for looking for macular edema in cases of wet macular degeneration or diabetic retinopathy. The OCT can also be used to map the optic nerve and is helpful for documenting and monitoring for glaucoma nerve damage (i.e., glaucomatous cupping).

ocular migraine. This is a migraine that either affects the vision (causing a migraine aura) or creates pain specifically in the eye. See migraine aura for more information on this topic.

Ocuflox. This is the trade name for the antibiotic eye drop ofloxacin. Ofloxacin is a moderately strong fluoroquinolone used for eye infections and prophylactic treatment after cataract surgery.

OCuSOFT. This is a brand of pre-made lid scrubs used for the treatment of blepharitis. These pre-moistened pads are used to gently clean debris off the eyelashes, improving lid hygiene, and making the eyes less irritable. These scrubs can sometimes be hard to find in stores, but are easily found online at Amazon.com. Other companies have begun making similar pads such as Systane Lid Wipes.

Ocuvite. This is an eye vitamin, produced by Bausch and Lomb, designed to decrease progression of aging changes from macular degeneration. This vitamin formula was created after the AREDS Study showed that certain antioxidants slowed the progression of macular degeneration changes in the retina. This original formula consisted of vitamins A (beta-carotene), C, E and the minerals zinc and copper. Since Bausch & Lomb helped supply the original formula (along with the

National Eye Institute), they immediately patented the combination and now sell the vitamin with a costly markup. Other companies have reached settlements with B&L and sell similar vitamins under different brands such as I-CAPS. Due to new research (and market pressures) the original formula is changing with the addition of lutein, zeaxanthin, and Omega-3 oils added to the mix. These additional supplements have been studied in the follow-up AREDS 2 Study.

ofloxacin. This is an antibiotic eye drop, also sold under the trade name Ocuflox. It is used for bacterial eye infections and often used as a prophylactic antibiotic before and after cataract surgery. This is a second generation fluoroquinolone similar to ciprofloxacin.

omega-3. These are fatty acids obtained from deep sea fish. There is some thought that Omega-3 supplements may help with macular degeneration, but they haven't been as beneficial as once hoped (see the AREDS 2 Study). Also, these fatty acids improve oil flow in the skin and may help with dry eye and the meibomian gland dysfunction found in blepharitis. The two types of Omega-3 acids most studied are the DHA and EPA variety. The best source is cold water fish such as salmon, tuna, herring, and (yuck) sardines. If you aren't a fish lover, omega-3s are available as supplements, both in oil and pill form. Vegetarians can get omega-3s from flaxseed, walnuts, and dark leafy vegetables.

Omnipred. This is the trade name for the steroid eye drop prednisolone acetate. Other names for this drop are Pred Forte and Econopred. This is a powerful topical steroid used to cool down inflammation. It is also used after cataract surgery to cool down inflammation and speed healing.

Opcon-A. This is an over-the-counter allergy drop used for itching and swelling of the eyelids. This drop is the same as the competing brand Naphcon-A. Opcon-A contains both an antihistamine and a vasoconstrictor. While effective for short term relief, I prefer the more powerful second generation allergy drops like Alaway/Zaditor and Patanol.

ophthalmologist. This is a doctor who treats medical eye problems and performs <u>laser</u> and eye surgery (like me). An ophthalmologist completes a four-year undergraduate degree with a focus on "pre-med" subjects including biology, chemistry, and physics. They then complete a four-year medical school program, working in a teaching hospital to become a medical doctor (MD). After this, we typically complete a year-long internship in a hospital rotating through inpatient wards, ICUs, and emergency rooms. We then proceed to an intense three-year residency eye program focusing on medical and surgical treatment of eye disease. Finally, some ophthalmologists take on an additional 1-2 years to sub-specialize in <u>retina</u>, <u>cornea</u>, <u>glaucoma</u>, etc.

optic disk. This is the insertion point of the optic nerve into the back of the eye. The <u>optic nerve</u> is a large nerve that connects the eyeball to the brain. This nerve inserts on the back of the eyeball and looks like a tube or pipe piercing the back of the eye. We can see the nerve insertion inside the eye during a dilated <u>retina</u> exam. Because we are viewing the nerve straight on it looks like a circle or a "disk" sitting in the middle of the retina. Examination of the disk is useful for monitoring many problems. For example, with <u>glaucoma</u> high ocular pressure slowly kills off the individual nerve fibers that fill the optic nerve. This creates a hollowed out area or "cup" that can be seen in the middle of the optic disk. This is called <u>glaucomatous cupping</u> and we follow the "cupping to disk ratio" over time to monitor for glaucoma damage. With <u>pseudotumor cerebri</u>, the pressure inside the skull (intracranial pressure) is high. This causes headaches and potentially neurologic problems if left untreated. The intracranial pressure is hard to measure, however, short of performing a spinal tap. However, this pressure can sometimes be seen at the optic disk because the fluid pressure can flow down the optic nerve and appear as optic disk swelling inside the eye.

optic nerve. The optic nerve is the large nerve that connects the eyeball to the brain. This nerve is actually comprised of over a million individual nerve fibers that send visual signals from the retina to the brain for processing. This nerve is obviously important and several eye diseases can affect it. The most common one is <u>glaucoma</u>. Glaucoma occurs when the internal eye pressure is too high, causing the death of the nerve fibers over time. Another optic nerve disorder we see is called optic neuritis. This is an inflammation of the optic nerve and is sometimes associated with multiple sclerosis (which causes inflammation of nerves in the brain as well). An ION (ischemic optic neuropathy) is like a mini-stroke to the optic nerve and occurs when the blood supply to the nerve is temporarily compromised. While most of the optic nerve is located behind the eyeball, a small portion can be seen from inside the eye as the optic disk.

optic nerve drusen. These are calcium crystals that form in the optic nerve and give the illusion of optic nerve swelling. The optic nerve is the large nerve that connects the eyeball to the brain. This nerve enters the back of the eye and this insertion can be seen inside the eye as the optic disk. Some people have natural calcium crystal deposits that form inside their optic disk. These calcium deposits are bulky, taking up space and giving the illusion of optic nerve swelling (papilledema). Swelling is a big deal as dangerous conditions like pseudotumor cerebri (high pressure inside the skull) can cause true optic nerve swelling. It is not always easy to differentiate between optic nerve drusen and true edema. In adults, drusen are easy to diagnose as the crystals glow and look like clusters of shiny rocks embedded in the nerve. In younger people the diagnoses is harder as the crystals are buried deeply and not as discernable. To truly detect optic nerve drusen, a number of tests can be performed. We can ultrasound the eye and look for the crystals - as the drusen are made of calcium, sound waves bounce off them and show up brightly on an ultrasound picture. A more invasive CAT scan can also be obtained as the crystals light up just like calcium-filled bones do. Another detection method is with a fluorescein angiogram. This test involves injection of a yellow dye into the blood stream to look for leakage inside the retina and optic nerve - calcium crystals don't leak fluid, while true optic nerve swelling does. While usually harmless, optic nerve drusen can cause problems with the peripheral vision, so a visual field test is sometimes obtained to establish a good baseline.

optic neuritis. This is an inflammation of the optic nerve that causes vision loss and occasionally eye pain. The optic nerve is the large nerve that connects the eye to the brain. Inflammation of this nerve will cause vision problems such as an enlarged blind spot and decreased vision. Optic neuritis occurs more in younger people (under 50) and is

sometimes a harbinger of more serious inflammatory nerve disorders like multiple sclerosis. Nerve swelling can sometimes be seen by the eye doctor by looking at the optic disk in the back of the eye. However, most of the optic nerve is located behind the eye and only a small portion of the nerve can actually be visualized during a dilated eye exam. Other hints of nerve swelling are pupil abnormalities and decreased color vision. More definitive diagnosis can be made by MRI, which is also useful for detecting other lesions in the brain consistent with multiple sclerosis. Treatment usually involves referral to a neurologist with possible IV steroids or other anti-inflammatory medicines. The vision usually comes back over a few weeks or months, though some permanent vision loss can occur.

optical coherence tomography.
An eye test that uses light waves to measure the surface of the retina ... similar to using sonar or ultrasound to measure the bottom of the ocean. See OCT for more information on this common test.

optician.
This is a person who fits and dispenses glasses and other corrective visual devices. Once you have a glasses prescription (from an optometrist or ophthalmologist) this is the person who actually measures your face and fits your glasses. They measure your pupillary distance, vertex distance, and determine where your bifocal should sit. They build the glasses and make sure they work properly.

Optivar.
This is the trade name for the antihistamine azelastine. This is a prescription allergy drop, used for itching and swelling of the eyes and eyelids. I've never prescribed this, given the ready supply of other allergy drops like Bepreve, Pataday and over-the-counter drops like Alaway/Zaditor.

optometrist.
A doctor of optometry specializes in primary eye care with a focus on refractive correction (glasses and contacts). These doctors typically complete a 4-year undergraduate degree, before going on to 4 more years of optometry graduate school. After this, an optometrist may go directly into practice or complete further residency

training if they have an interest in a specific fields of interest (like pediatrics or low-vision). An optometrist has an O.D. doctorate degree, and while they don't perform surgical procedures, they are licensed in most states to prescribe eye drop medications and therapeutic treatments. They are very good at optical correction and the fitting of challenging glasses and contact lenses. In many ways, the optometrist is like the "family practitioner" of the eye world - they are often the first person to detect new eye problems and will refer medical/surgical problems to the appropriate ophthalmologist (general or sub-specialist) when warranted.

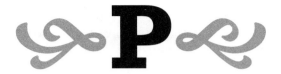

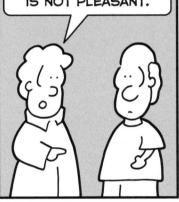

THE TREATMENT FOR MACULAR DEGENERATION IS NOT PLEASANT.

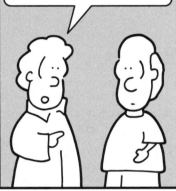

BUT AT LEAST IT'S BETTER THAN A SHARP STICK IN THE EYE.

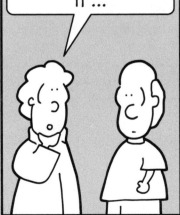

ACTUALLY, COME TO THINK OF IT ...

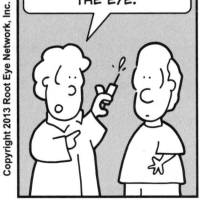

... THE TREATMENT IS <u>EXACTLY</u> LIKE A SHARP STICK IN THE EYE.

www.RootEyeDictionary.com

Copyright 2013 Root Eye Network, Inc.

pachymetry. This is the measurement of corneal thickness. The cornea is the clear window that makes up the front of the eye and allows light to enter the eye. The corneal thickness is an important measurement for a couple of reasons. An abnormally thin or thick cornea can affect pressure measurements when screening for glaucoma. With LASIK eye surgery, some of the cornea is removed with a laser in order to change the focus of the eye ... if your cornea is too thin to begin with, you might not be a good candidate for LASIK. We measure the cornea with a machine called a "pachymeter" ... it is a small ultrasonic probe that briefly touches the surface of the anesthetized eye. It only takes a few seconds to obtain this measurement and the process is painless. Corneal thickness is a relatively stable measurement and rarely changes with time unless you have problems with corneal swelling such as from Fuchs' dystrophy.

papilledema. This is bilateral swelling of the optic nerves secondary to high intracranial pressure. The brain sits inside the skull and is suspended by membranes, floating in fluid. This fluid is the cerebral spinal fluid (CSF) and is similar to the aqueous fluid in the eyeball itself. If the pressure of this CSF is high, such as in pseudotumor cerebri, this can cause headaches and neurologic changes. Unfortunately, it is very hard to actually measure the pressure inside the skull. One could always drill a hole through the skull and see how fast the water comes out, but for obvious reasons this is not feasible. Instead, a spinal tap is performed. A needle is inserted in the lower back. Since the fluid in the spine is connected to the brain, a neurologist can estimate the brain pressure by measuring the "opening pressure" during the spinal tap. This is not fun either, but is really the only way to truly know the brain pressure. Fortunately, an eye doctor can sometimes estimate the CSF pressure by dilating the eye and looking at the optic disk. The eyeball is a direct extension of the brain ... and the pressure from the brain fluid will travel down the optic nerves and be visible as swelling inside the eye. This swelling is called papilledema. If the pressure is high enough, the nerves will swell and elevate like a volcano, causing blurring of the normally crisp nerve margins.

papilloma. A papilloma is a bump on the eyelid or skin around the eye that looks like a skin tag. These are almost always harmless proliferations of skin cells that have a stuck-on appearance and can be very unsightly. They typically form on the skin around the eyelids and even along the lid margin in the eyelash line. They are sometimes caused by the human papilloma virus (like a wart) but usually they have no known cause. A papilloma can usually be taken off in the office by numbing the skin and cutting them off at the base. Cautery (with a surgical "soldering iron") is usually performed at the base to stop bleeding and to decrease the chance of the papilloma coming back. Cautery gives a surprisingly good cosmetic result, though we have to be careful when working near the edge of the eyelid. If the papilloma is in the lash line, there is a chance that the lashes will not regrow in that spot or they may grow in a funny direction when the area heals (this is called trichiasis).

Pataday. A prescription strength allergy drop that is good for treating itching and swelling around the eyes. This medicine's claim-to-fame is that it is a once-a-day drop. Similar strength allergy drops include Bepreve and Lastacaft.

Patanol. One of the more powerful allergy drops. It is good for itching and swelling around the eyes. This is a prescription medication that has been supplanted by Pataday (which has twice the active ingredient).

patching. Patching an eye shut is useful for several conditions. The most common one is amblyopia, where an eye becomes "lazy" from disuse in childhood. A patch is used to cover the good eye and force the "lazy" eye to work better. Patching is also used for therapeutic effect in cases of eye pain. If you are having extraordinary eye pain from a corneal abrasion the eye can be patched shut. However, I typically avoid prolonged patching in an eye that has an active infection, as bacteria like warm, dark places. Patching can also be useful when an eye won't shut. For example, after retrobulbar block anesthesia (used for difficult or prolonged eye surgery), the eye will not close all the way for several hours. To keep the eye from drying out, the eye is patched shut overnight.

PD. This stands for "pupillary distance," which is the distance between the pupils of each eye. This is an important measurement used in the creation of glasses. See pupillary distance for a more detailed explanation.

phacoemulsification. This is the modern surgical technique for removing cataracts by breaking apart (emulsifying) the lens with ultrasonic vibrations. During cataract surgery, the cloudy lens is removed from the eye. To pull this off, the surgeon first breaks the lens into tiny pieces before vacuuming it out. This is accomplished with a phacoemulsification probe. This ultrasonic technique is a huge improvement as it allows cataract surgery to be performed through a quickly healing microincision. The underlying technology behind phacoemulsification has drastically improved over the past three decades, with less and less energy being required to get the job done. Less energy means safer surgery and quicker healing times. Attempts at using lasers to break up cataracts are being studied, but this hasn't yet been found to work as well.

phakic. A term used to describe an eye that has its natural lens still in place. This is opposed to the term "pseudophakic," which is a person who has a plastic implant in their eye (such as after cataract surgery). If a person has NO lens in their eye (neither their natural lens or cataract implant), we would call this person "aphakic." Aphakia is rare these days, and usually only occurs after trauma or difficulties with prior cataract surgery where a new lens couldn't be implanted.

pheniramine. This is a generic antihistamine drug found in many over-the-counter allergy drops such as Opcon-A and Naphcon-A. While effective, this antihistamine is not as powerful as more modern drugs like ketotifen (found in Alaway and Zaditor) and Pataday.

phenylephrine. This is a dilating drop used during an eye exam to better view the retina. This drop works by stimulating the sympathetic system in order to dilate the pupil. It doesn't cause cycloplegia so there is less problems with blurry vision when dilated. However, this drop does not dilate the pupil enough when used by itself, so it's usually used in

conjunction with a cycloplegic like tropicamide. This medication is now being used in over-the-counter decongestants like Sudafed as a replacement for the original pseudoephedrine (which you have to sign for to insure you are not a methamphetamine junkie).

phoropter. This is the machine we use to check your glasses prescription. It is filled with lenses that we flip in front of your eyes, saying "one or two" the whole time as you read the eye chart. The phoropter is the best way to refine an eyeglass prescription, as we can use this machine to detect and fix your astigmatism as well. Unfortunately, some of our patients can't use the phoropter machine because it requires a certain amount of subjective feedback. Young children and the infirm may need to be checked with less precise measurements such as the retinoscope.

photophobia. This is a fancy way of saying pain or sensitivity to light. When an eye is irritated, the iris muscle inside the eye becomes sensitive. The iris is the colored part of our eye - it is a round muscle that dilates and constricts the pupil to control the amount of light entering the eye. This muscle can become inflamed and hurts. With bright lights, the muscle "spasms" and hurts even more. Photophobia can be treated by dilating the eye with cycloplegic eye drops. These drops dilate the pupil, but they also temporarily "paralyze" the iris muscle so it won't spasm. It is like "paralyzing" a broken leg - by immobilizing it in a cast, you don't walk on it, and thus it won't hurt as much. If you are experiencing new photophobia, you should see your eye doctor to insure you don't have a corneal abrasion or more serious internal ocular inflammation such as uveitis.

photoreceptors. After light enters the eye it eventually strikes the retina, which works like the film in a camera. The photoreceptors are the cells within the retina that actually detect light photons and convert them into a signal our body can detect. These photoreceptors come in different varieties. Cones are the cells that detect color and are especially important for our daylight and fine central vision. Rods can only see in black and white, but are highly sensitive and important for night vision and our peripheral vision.

pilocarpine. This is a pupil-constricting eye drop. Pilocarpine has been around for a long time and it makes the pupil constrict by stimulating the iris muscles to contract. In the eye doctor's office, pilocarpine is often used immediately prior to SLT or ALT laser therapy. Pilocarpine is effective in lowering eye pressure, though it is no longer first-line therapy for glaucoma because of the visual side effects (small pupils can make the vision a little blurry).

pinguecula. This is a white or yellow "bump" seen on the white part of the eye. The entire eye is covered by a very thin layer of skin called the conjunctiva. This conjunctiva is very delicate and thin. In fact, you can see red blood vessels coursing through this skin by looking in the mirror. The conjunctiva protects the eye but can become irritated by constant wind and sun exposure. When the skin is irritated, it tends to thicken and become discolored (like a callus on the hand or foot). This creates a discolored bump on the eye. A pinguecula can become irritated and make the eye sensitive. Treatment is usually with artificial tears and sparing use of mild steroid. On rare occasions, surgical excision can be considered, but most pinguecula are mild and only a minor cosmetic nuisance.

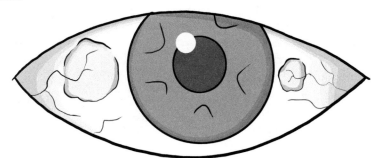

A pinguecula looks like an elevated, yellowish
bump on the white of the eye.

pinhole. When we are checking your vision in our office, one of the most common tests we perform is called the "pinhole test." After you read the eye chart wearing your glasses, we recheck your vision while you look through a plastic patch that has little holes punched through it. Many people will actually see better when looking through the pinholes ... reading several lines lower on the eye chart. This pinhole improvement is usually an indicator that your glasses need to be updated. The pinhole test works because it turns your eye from a "focusing telescope" system into a simple "pinhole camera." Pinhole cameras have no lenses and don't need to be focused like a traditional camera ... by letting light into the camera through a tiny pinhole, the image is always in focus. Many small cameras, such as the one in your cell phone, use a pinhole and require little focusing. The eye is much larger, however, and needs to be focused like a telescope. The pinhole test is pretty cool, but unfortunately we can't make your glasses this way as the pinhole effect is pretty dim and would really mess up your peripheral vision. However, if you ever find yourself on a deserted island and the natives steal your glasses, you may be able to construct your own pinhole glasses out of shells or leaves and see well enough to survive! If this happens and you make it back alive ... please let me know and consider adding me to your will.

pink eye. This is a descriptive term for conjunctivitis. The majority of conjunctivitis cases are caused by viral infection (as opposed to allergic or bacterial infection) so the term "pink eye" is more commonly used to describe <u>viral conjunctivitis</u>. See the <u>conjunctivitis</u> entry for more information.

Plaquenil. Plaquenil (hydroxychloroquine) is an anti-inflammatory medication that is commonly used in cases of rheumatoid arthritis and lupus. It was originally (and still) used as an anti-malaria drug but has also been found to decrease inflammation in the body. While very effective, this medication can have ocular side effects. Prolonged use can lead to pigmentary changes in the <u>retina</u> and create central vision loss. The vision loss can be detected using a <u>visual field</u> testing machine that focuses on the central 10 degrees of your vision. Color vision seems to be affected first, so often this test is performed with a red filter. As damage occurs, the retina can develop a classic "bulls eye" appearance that can be seen on a dilated eye exam. Despite the potential risk, these visual problems are extremely rare and seem to present more with higher dosages of medicine taken for many years. The longer you are on Plaquenil, the more important regular eye checkups become.

pneumatic retinopexy. This is a procedure used to repair a retinal detachment using a gas bubble. With a <u>retinal detachment</u>, the <u>retina</u> peels off the back of the eye like wallpaper peeling off a wall. To help reapproximate the retina into its normal position, a gas bubble can be injected into the eye. This pushes the retina back in place, holding it down and allowing retinal breaks/holes to be sealed with <u>laser</u> or cryotherapy (cold probe). The benefit to a pneumatic treatment is that it can be performed in the <u>retina specialist's</u> office without requiring surgery. The downside is that this procedure only works if the retina tear is small and located at the top of the eye (because gas bubbles float upwards). Also, the pneumatic retinopexy doesn't always work, and may still require additional retinal surgeries such as <u>vitrectomy</u> or <u>scleral buckle</u> procedure.

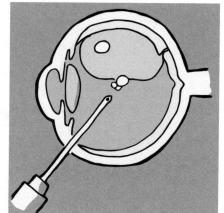

With a pneumatic retinopexy, gas floats and holds
the detached retina in place.

POAG. This is the abbreviation for Primary Open Angle Glaucoma. This is the type of glaucoma that most people have, where the eye pressure is chronically elevated leading to gradual <u>optic nerve</u> damage. See <u>chronic open angle glaucoma</u> (COAG) for more details on this topic.

polymyxin. An antibiotic found in combination with other medications such as in <u>Neosporin</u>, <u>Polysporin</u>, and <u>Polytrim</u>.

polymyxin Sulfate/TMP. This is a combination <u>antibiotic</u> drop. The trade name for this combination is <u>Polytrim</u>. This drop is now generic and inexpensive. Long-term use can be irritating to the <u>cornea</u>, however.

Polysporin. This is a combination <u>antibiotic</u> eye drop containing <u>bacitracin</u> and <u>polymyxin</u>. This drug is similar to <u>Neosporin</u>, except that neomycin has been removed (many people have a sensitivity to neomycin).

Polytrim. This is a combination <u>antibiotic</u> eye drop containing <u>polymyxin</u> and trimethoprim. It is available as an inexpensive generic.

polyvinyl alcohol. A synthetic lubricant used in many <u>rewetting</u> <u>drops</u>. It is safe and non-toxic, but has a terrible sounding name if you ask me ... who wants to put poly, vinyl, or alcohol in their eye, after all?

Pred-Forte. A popular <u>steroid</u> eye drop. Pred-Forte is the trade name for <u>prednisolone</u> acetate. Steroid eye drops are good at cooling down ocular inflammation caused by <u>iritis</u> or <u>uveitis</u>. This drop is commonly used after <u>cataract surgery</u>, as well, to speed recovery.

prednisolone. Prednisolone acetate is the most common <u>steroid</u> drop we use for the eye. This comes under the trade names <u>Pred-Forte</u> and <u>Econopred</u>. Steroid drops are used to cool down inflammation and are often used after <u>cataract surgery</u>.

presbyopia. This is the process by which you become more reliant on <u>reading glasses</u> as you get older. When we are born, we have a clear <u>lens</u> that sits inside our eye. This lens is flexible and can change shape to help us focus. The lens can "flatten" like a pancake and allow a child to see a distant mountain, or the lens can "round out" like a marble and allow a child to focus on extremely close objects such as a butterfly landing on the nose. This lens shaping ability is called "accommodation." As we get older, the lens begins to stiffen a little bit and doesn't go "round" as easily as it used to. Once we hit 40 years of age, the lens is so rigid that we have a hard time reading things close-up and find ourselves holding books further and further away. As the lens continues to harden we require bifocals or reading glasses for near tasks. This process of lens stiffening and the loss of focal range is called presbyopia and is a normal aging change in our eye.

PreserVision. This is an eye vitamin designed to decrease the progression of macular degeneration. This brand is produced by Bausch & Lomb, but differs from their original Ocuvite product in that the pills are smaller and easier to swallow. The packaging for eye vitamins keeps changing, but as long as you take an AREDS (or AREDS 2) formulation, you should be fine. Remember smokers ... look on the back of the packaging to make sure there isn't any beta-carotene in the vitamins you buy, as this vitamin may increase your risk of lung cancer.

pressure. In regards to the eye, "pressure" usually refers to the intraocular pressure - the pressure inside the eyeball itself. Eye pressure can be measured a number of ways, but all of the methods involve pushing on the eye to estimate the pressure within. This is akin to kicking a car tire with your foot in order to estimate the internal tire pressure. In a doctor's office, pressure is usually measured with applanation tonometry. This is a blue light attached to a weighted mechanism that pushes on the surface of the cornea. Topical numbing drops are used, so the process is quick and painless. Another method to measure pressure is with a hand-held Tono-Pen device. This is an electronic gadget that looks like a large pen or marker and is used to measure the pressure electronically. The Tono-Pen is not terribly accurate, but sometimes it is the only way to check pressure in patients who can't get into the microscope or are bedridden. The final way to check pressure, and the one you may be most familiar with, is the "air puff." This device puffs air at the cornea and measures the surface distortion caused by the shockwave. The air puff is used in some eye offices because it requires little skill to learn and is easy to keep sterile. It is seldom used in medical ophthalmology, however, as the puff is uncomfortable and the measurements may not be as accurate as applanation tonometry (though this is highly debated by some). On our scale, "normal" eye pressure is 10-21, with distribution being skewed toward the higher pressures.   High eye pressure is associated with glaucoma and can also be present with inflammation or bleeding inside the eye (from traumatic or after surgery). Low pressure can be seen with wound leaks after surgery and sometimes with internal inflammation like uveitis.

prism. This is a lens ground into a pair of glasses that is designed to bend light and help alleviate double vision. With double vision (also known as diplopia), people see two of the same object. This is usually because of an alignment problem between the eyes such as when someone is cross-eyed. To help alleviate this doubling, prism correction can be ground into a pair of spectacles to bend the light in such a way that the doubling goes back to "normal." Prism glasses are effective for many people, but they have some limitations. Prism adds significant thickness and cost to the glasses. They are also difficult to get "just right" and may require many visits and possible remakes (frustrating for both the patient and the optical shop).   Also, some people have alignment problems that vary throughout the day ... they may seem fine in the morning, but as the day progresses their double vision worsens. Prism glasses don't work well in this situation as the correction needed is constantly changing.   Finally, some people have double vision that is more pronounced at distance, or near, or when looking in a particular direction. Once again, prism glasses can only correct a 'single' alignment problem and so several pairs of glasses may be required (such as separate distance and reading glasses).

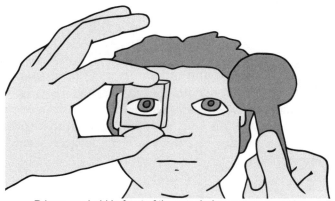

Prisms are held in front of the eye during an eye exam to eliminate diplopia (double vision).

PRK. This stands for "photorefractive keratectomy" and is a laser procedure similar to LASIK used to correct refractive problems like nearsightedness. Like LASIK, an excimer laser is used to sculpt and resurface the shape of the cornea. With LASIK, however, a partial thickness flap is created and flipped up before applying the laser treatment. This flap is then laid back into place and results in more comfort and quicker healing time. With PRK, however, there is no flap and the laser ablation is performed on the surface of the cornea itself. This results in a large corneal abrasion, with more discomfort and a slower healing time than LASIK. PRK is a good option for people with thinner corneas who are not good candidates for the more popular LASIK procedure.

progressive lenses. These are "no line" bifocals. They look like normal glasses, but the further you look down the stronger the bifocal "progressively" becomes. This type of bifocal is useful for active people because you can literally tilt your head to appropriately focus on different objects. For example, you might look through the top part of the progressive to see your car speedometer, and look further down to see your phone. Progressives aren't for everyone, however. Some people don't like them because the bottom part of the glass seems distorted when walking around. Also, the "sweet spot" for crisp reading vision is much smaller than a traditional bifocal, which can be annoying for long periods of reading. They also cost a little more than a traditional bifocal or trifocal. There are several brands of progressive lenses, but generally the Varilux brand is the highest quality model that seems to provide the most comfort for a majority of users.

Prolensa. This is an anti-inflammatory eye drop (an NSAID medication) that is commonly used after cataract surgery to decrease irritation and inflammation. This medicine contains the same medication (bromfenac) as Bromday but with a slightly decreased concentration of the active ingredient. I mainly use this medicine to decrease the chance of retinal swelling after surgery.

proparacaine. This is an <u>anesthetic drop</u> using during an eye exam. This drop numbs the corneal nerves and makes it easier to perform <u>applanation tonometry</u> (<u>pressure</u> checking). We also use this drop before any procedures near the eye, such as <u>foreign body</u> removal. Another drop we use is <u>tetracaine</u>, though we prefer proparacaine in the office as it stings less going in. There aren't really any home applications with this medication ... while it does help with pain, the duration is short (10-20 minutes). Repeated applications of anesthetic are toxic to the <u>cornea</u> and will keep a wound (such as a <u>corneal abrasion</u>) from healing.

proptosis. This is when the eye bulges out. The eye sits inside the eye socket like a scoop of ice cream sitting inside a waffle cone. When the contents of the eye socket swell, there is not a lot of room to expand except forward, so the eye tends to protrude outwards. Proptosis of the eye can occur for many reasons, though the most common is secondary to <u>thyroid eye disease</u> (i.e., <u>Graves' disease</u>) which causes the eye muscles behind the eye to enlarge over time. There are more concerning causes for proptosis, including inflammation, infection, and neoplastic processes (i.e., a tumor). Proptosis needs to be evaluated in the office to rule out these dangerous conditions. Often a CT ("CAT scan") is ordered.

prostaglandin. This is a class of medications used for treating <u>glaucoma</u>. The prostaglandins work by increasing outflow of <u>aqueous</u> fluid from the eye. Examples include <u>Xalatan</u> (<u>latanoprost</u>), <u>Travatan</u> (<u>travoprost</u>), and <u>Lumigan</u> (<u>bimatoprost</u>). These medications are typically dosed once a day. The main complication of these drops is eye redness and irritation, which is why most people take their drops at bedtime so they can sleep through this redness. Other side effects include <u>eyelash</u> growth (woman tend to like this) and pigmentary changes to the skin and iris. All of these findings are quite rare, and prostaglandin drops work so well that they are initial therapy for most people with a new diagnosis of glaucoma. Xalatan was the first prostaglandin eye drop in use - it is now available as generic latanoprost, making this therapy even more affordable.

PRP. This stands for panretinal photocoagulation, and is a <u>laser</u> treatment commonly used for <u>diabetic retinopathy</u>. With diabetes, blood vessels become leaky and the retinal tissue in the eye can become hungry for oxygen because of poor blood delivery. The oxygen-starved retina cells respond by producing protective hormones called <u>VEGF</u> (vascular endothelial growth factor). VEGF causes the formation of new blood vessels, which at first glance ought to be a good idea ... after all, new blood vessels might help feed the hungry <u>retina</u>! Unfortunately, the new blood vessels are abnormal and tend to scar, contract, and bleed easily. This can lead to <u>retinal detachments</u> and <u>vitreous hemorrhage</u>. The abnormal blood vessels can even grow into the <u>trabecular meshwork</u> (the "drain" of the eye) similar to tree roots growing into a house's plumbing. This can lead to <u>acute glaucoma</u> with severe vision loss. This abnormal vessel growth is called <u>neovascularization</u> and it needs to be treated before it gets out of hand. To treat neovascularization, a PRP laser procedure is performed. With this procedure, hundreds (sometimes thousands) of laser spots are burned into the peripheral retina, essentially destroying the peripheral retinal cells. By sacrificing the hungry peripheral retina (where most of the oxygen deprivation is occurring) less VEGF is produced and the neovascularization will stop and even regress. While it may seem barbaric to sacrifice part of the retina in this fashion, the procedure is very important as it saves the more important central vision. Few people notice visual changes after the PRP procedure ... though some complain of a decrease in night vision.

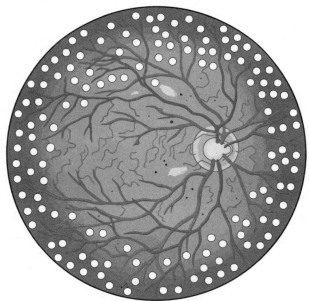

PRP laser spots are applied to the retinal periphery in an attempt
to protect the important central vision.

pseudoexfoliation.

Pseudoexfoliation syndrome is a common ocular finding, especially if you are of Scandinavian descent. With this condition, a flaky dandruff-like material forms on the surface of your lens/cataract. This material rubs off over a lifetime and can cause glaucoma if the material "clogs the drain" inside your eye. This material also forms on the support strings that hold your lens in position behind your iris. These strings are called zonules, and surround the cataract/lens in a 360-degree ring like springs on a trampoline. With pseudoexfoliation syndrome, the flaky material weakens these springs. If the zonular springs break during surgery, the cataract can fall into the back of the eye and will require removal by a retina specialist (a second operation). We can detect pseudoexfoliation during a routine eye exam.

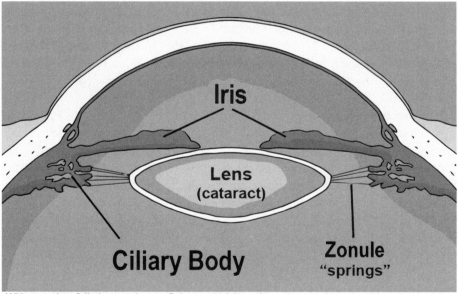

With pseudoexfoliation syndrome, flakey material weakens the zonule springs that suspend the lens inside the eye. This can cause the lens to dislocate during cataract surgery.

pseudomonas.

This is a water-borne bacteria that commonly sticks to contact lenses and can cause a corneal ulcer. Pseudomonas is the same bacteria that causes "swimmer's ear" and it tends to proliferate in watery environments (such as contact lens solution and within contacts themselves). If this bacteria colonizes the cornea, it can cause a bad corneal ulcer. Pseudomonas infection can be challenging to treat as it tends to be resistant to many of the older antibiotics. For this reason, any infection related to contact lens use needs to be evaluated by an eye doctor and treated with aggressive antibiotics.

pseudophakic. A medical term used to describe an eye that has already had <u>cataract surgery</u> and now contains a plastic or "pseudo" lens <u>implant</u>. Compare this to the term "<u>phakic</u>" (an eye that contains its natural lens) or "<u>aphakic</u>" (an eye that has no lens at all).

pseudotumor cerebri. This is when the pressure inside the cranial cavity (i.e., inside the skull) is too high. The brain sits inside the skull and is suspended in a bath of fluid called the CSF (cerebrospinal fluid). This fluid cushions the brain and keeps it buoyant inside this cramped space. This fluid is constantly being renewed and reabsorbed back into the body. If the drainage of CSF fluid is blocked for some reason, the pressure inside the skull will increase. This creates headaches, and if severe and long-lasting, can create long-term neurologic and visual changes that may be permanent. Pseudotumor cerebri (also called idiopathic intracranial hypertension) can occur for many reasons, such as a reaction to antibiotics, hormonal changes, or a temporary thrombosis of the draining veins inside the skull. We see it most often in younger women of child-bearing years who've gained a little weight recently. Initial diagnosis is often made by an eye doctor as the fluid pressure can transmit to the back of the eye and be seen as swelling of the <u>optic nerve</u> (<u>papilledema</u>) during a dilated eye exam. More definitive diagnosis is made with a spinal tap to measure the "opening pressure." Treatment is first geared at finding the underlying cause. This may involve evaluation with a neurologist and an MRI of the head to look for vein thrombosis. If no obvious cause is found, treatment begins with the oral pill <u>Diamox</u>. This is a water pill that decreases the production of CSF fluid and can lower CSF pressure. Weight loss is also a key in treatment. Sometimes, only a 5 to 10 percent reduction in weight can produce a dramatic improvement in symptoms. If the high pressure continues, then a neurosurgeon may need to insert a surgical drain to remove the excess fluid away from the brain.

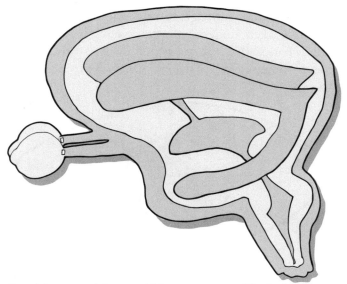

Pseudotumor cerebri causes high pressure around the brain. This pressure can press on the optic nerves at the back of the eyes.

pterygium. This is a small yellow-white growth that forms on the eye, starting from the white conjunctival skin, and spreading over the clear cornea. These are harmless growths and common in people with sun exposure or who work outside. The <u>conjunctiva</u> is a very thin layer of skin that covers the eye. This skin can become irritated by a lifetime of sun and wind exposure, causing the skin to thicken and grow a little bit … just like chronic irritation will cause the thickening of skin elsewhere on the body such as a callus on the hands or feet. When skin thickening happens on the eye, we call this a pterygium (or <u>pinguecula</u> if the spot is isolated on the conjunctiva only). Pterygium only occurs on the white of the eye at the three and nine o'clock positions because this is the part of the eye exposed to the elements (i.e., not covered by the <u>eyelids</u>). A pterygium can be aggravating as the eyelid rubs over it with every blink. When irritated, the pterygium can swell, turn red, and cause even more eye irritation. Early treatment usually involves lubrication with <u>artificial tears</u> and sunglasses. If this is not helping, <u>allergy drops</u> and even a mild <u>steroid</u> can be used to cool the eye down. <u>Visine</u> can be used as a short-term solution but should be used sparingly. If the pterygium persists, gets larger, or approaches the visual axis, than surgical excision can be considered. There are many techniques for removing a pterygium but the most definitive is a "conjunctival autograph." This involves cutting the pterygium off and sewing/grafting another piece of conjunctival tissue (harvested from underneath the eyelid) in its place. This vastly decreases the chance that the pterygium will reform in the future and gives a good cosmetic result. This is done under topical anesthesia in the operating room.

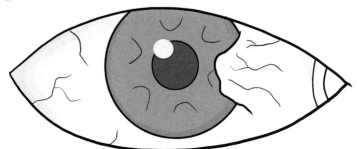

A pterygium looks like a fleshy bump growing over the colored part of the eye.

ptosis. A fancy way to say "droopy eyelid." Ptosis means that the edge of the upper <u>eyelid</u> is actually dropping down, sometimes bad enough to cover the <u>pupil</u> and obstruct vision. Many people with ptosis find themselves tilting their head back or constantly raising their eyebrows in order to lift their eyelids up and see properly. Ptosis can be caused by many things, including congenital ptosis, traumatic injury and neuromuscular disorders like <u>myasthenia gravis</u>. Eyelid drooping can also occur from age stretching of the muscle that holds the eyelid open. Treatment involves surgical tightening of the eyelid retractor muscle. When people describe their eye as drooping, they aren't always talking about ptosis ... most people actually have <u>dermatochalasis</u>. This is when the skin above the eye becomes lax and droops down over the eyelashes. This is completely different and easier to treat with a <u>blepharoplasty</u> (a surgery to remove this excess skin).

puncta. This is a small drainage hole located on the inner <u>eyelid</u> that drains excess tears into the nose. Normally, the <u>tear film</u> is generated from the inner eyelids and washes down the surface of the eye like a waterfall. The fluid then forms a small "lake" along the lower eyelid. Tears from this lake drain through the punctum (the plural of puncta) and into a drainage canal under the skin. Eventually, the tears flow down the nasolacrimal duct and empty out into the nose. This pathway explains why people with runny eyes often have a runny nose as well. Some people have a problem with their puncta working correctly. Their puncta may be too small or may have been scarred shut from chronic lid irritation. Aging can cause the lower lid to loosen and rotate outwards so that the puncta is no longer able to reach the tear film at all. Some of these drainage problems can be fixed with surgery (but not easily). Puncta blockage is sometimes a good thing - with dry eye we occasionally block the puncta with temporary punctal plugs and we can even close the puncta permanently using cautery.

punctal occlusion.
This is a technique used to decrease the absorption of eye drop medications. Normally when you put eye drops in, the medication drains through the puncta, down the nasolacrimal duct, and into the nose. This is why people have a runny nose when their eyes are teary. Unfortunately, the nose absorbs medicines directly into the blood stream (which is why cocaine is snorted and not swallowed). Some of the medicines we use can have significant systemic absorption and can cause side effects. Overall these side effects are rare, but you can perform punctal occlusion to help avoid the absorption. After you put your eye drops in, immediately close your eyes. Don't blink, as blinking can act as a pump and shoot the medicine right into your nose. Instead, take your fingers and press the bridge of your nose right next to your eyes. Hold this for a good 20 seconds and this will decrease your systemic nose absorption significantly.

punctal plugs.
These are small silicone devices inserted into the puncta drainage holes in the eye to allow the tears to last longer and help correct dry eye. Punctal plugs are relatively easy to insert and this can be done right in the exam chair. By slowing down the tear drainage, the ocular surface is better moistened. The plugs are microscopic and can't be easily seen or felt. Unfortunately, the plugs have a tendency to fall out ... this can occur weeks or months after insertion, though I've seen plugs last as long as 10 years in good position. Occasionally, the plugs themselves cause mild irritation and excessive tearing - in these cases we simply remove the plugs using tweezers. More permanent closure of the puncta can be done, but I prefer to use the silicone plugs because they can always be removed later if needed.

pupil. The pupil is the black circle in the middle of the eye. It is actually a hole in the middle of the iris that allows light to enter the back of the eye. The size of the pupil is controlled by the iris muscle in response to ambient lighting. In dark rooms, the pupil enlarges to allow more light to strike the retina. Conversely, in well-lit rooms the pupil constricts to protect the retina and to make the vision look crisper. While the pupil is normally round, there are some conditions that can make the pupil oddly shaped. For example, inflammation of the iris (iritis) can make the pupil edge "stick" to the lens underneath, causing the pupil shape to distort. This distortion is called iris synechiae.

pupillary distance. The pupillary distance is the measured distance between the pupils of both your eyes. When glasses are made, they need to be created to correct for your eye separation. Some people have wide-set eyes and other have near-set eyes, so this can vary widely. This measurement is made by your optician after you pick a new glasses frame, and the measurement is used when your lenses are cut and fitted into the frame. Normally, your "PD" measurement is not measured by your optometrist/ophthalmologist during a clinic visit and so is not written on a glasses prescription (and thus is not part of your medical records). There is a good reason for this - glass "fitting measurements" need to be made by the same person who actually constructs your glasses and the proper fitting of glasses is somewhat dependent upon what frame and glasses style you are actually buying. Some people would like to obtain their PD measurement so they can order glasses online, as overseas spectacles can be found for surprisingly low cost. Local opticians don't like to measure the pupillary distance and just "give out" this measurement for someone else to use. In fact, in some states, they aren't allowed to as it would make them responsible for the glasses (no matter who made them). This reticence on the part of local opticians is not from "greed" or "obstinance," but an attempt to avoid the inevitable backlash from angry online customers. Online glasses are often made to substandard standards in Indonesia/China with lower quality frames. These glasses can be uncomfortable or cause eye strain because of incorrectly cut PD correction and a poor-fitting frame. Also, foreign producers don't measure your vertex distance (the distance from the eye to the back of the glass), bifocal segment height, or adjust your progressive lens placement. If a customer receives a pair of crummy glasses in the mail, there is no easy way to "fix" them online ... so the only recourse is to return to the local optical shop to complain and try to get them adjusted or remade. This creates unnecessary contention between the customer and optical workers who end up spending inordinate amounts of time trying to fix crummy glasses for free that they didn't even make (glasses that might even break during the adjustment process with no way to replace them). This situation is comparable to seeing a local tailor/dressmaker and getting measurements for a dress/tuxedo, ordering an outfit from China, and then complaining to your local tailor/dressmaker when it doesn't fit well. Poorly fit mail-order glasses are more common if you have a "strong" glasses prescription or finicky bifocal requirements. Some people have great success with online sellers, but buyer beware. It is always safer to get your glasses locally ... even if you have to shop around a little to find acceptable costs. This way you can try on the frame to get one that is comfortable, get your eyes measured by the shop that actually uses their own measurements, and have them adjusted afterwards (or even completely remade if necessary) without feeling guilty.

PVD. This is the abbreviation for posterior vitreous detachment. See vitreous detachment for more information on this common cause of flashes and floaters.

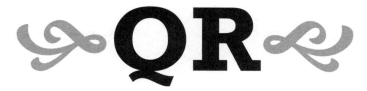

QR

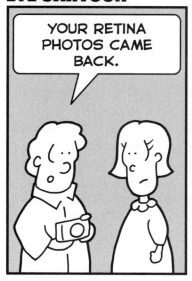

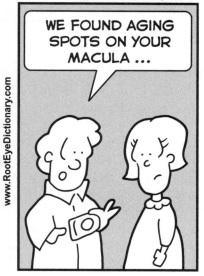

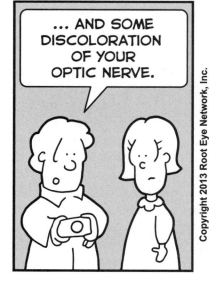

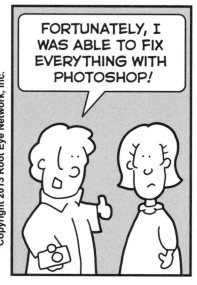

www.RootEyeDictionary.com

Copyright 2013 Root Eye Network, Inc.

radial keratotomy. Also called "RK," this is an older refractive surgery style in which a diamond knife is used to make radial cuts in the cornea. These incisions change the shape of the cornea and can correct nearsightedness. This technique was invented by a Russian ophthalmologist in the '70s and was very popular in the '80s and early '90s. While effective, some people with RK continue to have corneal shape fluctuations decades later and go on to become farsighted. While a successful procedure, this technique has since been supplanted by more predictable laser procedures like LASIK and PRK.

reading glasses. These are glasses that are focused for viewing near objects ... such as when reading a book. Inexpensive, over-the-counter reading glasses work well for many people and range in diopter power from weak +1.00 glass, all the way up to +3.50 readers. The power of your "cheaters" depends upon your age and how close you like to hold books to your face. If you have significant refractive error (nearsightedness, farsightedness, or astigmatism) you may require prescription reading glasses (or a bifocal) for best vision. Also, keep in mind that cheap OTC reading glasses are designed to fit the average person ... if your eyes are narrow or wide-set, they may not be as comfortable or clear as a custom glass. Your need for reading glasses occurs because of presbyopia (aging changes inside the eye), and is normal after the age of forty.

recurrent erosion. This is a corneal abrasion that recurs because it doesn't "heal right," kind of like a skin cut that keeps reopening. The cornea is the clear structure that lies at the front of the eye, forming the ocular surface that allows light to enter the eye. The cornea is relatively tough but it is covered by a more delicate layer of skin called the corneal "epithelium." The corneal skin is thin and can easily rub or scratch off due to trauma or abrasion caused by a piece of sand in the eye. Surface scratches are called "corneal abrasions" and can cause much discomfort. A recurrent erosion occurs when the epithelial skin doesn't heal well enough to the cornea. Repeated blinking can cause the corneal epithelium to scratch off again. This usually happens in the morning when the eyes are most dry. When the eyes pop open, the suction pulls off the epithelium again. This repetitive process can make the erosion take forever to heal. You can almost imagine that the surface epithelium is like a carpet that grows back over a concrete foundation. With recurrent erosion, the concrete gets "sandy" or "rough" in one spot such that carpet has a hard time tacking down in that particular area. Treatment for a recurrent erosion usually begins with aggressive night-time lubrication and ointments but can expand to include night-time patching and bandage <u>contact</u> lenses. If these aren't working, more aggressive surgical treatments can be considered, such as polishing the underlying cornea with a diamond burr or stromal puncture (using a needle to create small divots in the cornea for the surface epithelium to grow down into and stick better).

refraction. This is the method used to determine someone's <u>glasses prescription</u>. Most refraction is performed with a <u>phoropter</u>. This is the optical device you look through while reading an eye chart - it contains lenses and can be used to determine your <u>refractive error</u> (nearsightedness and farsightedness) and correct <u>astigmatism</u>. Refraction requires feedback from our patients, so this technique can be especially tough in children and in non-verbal people (ex.: dementia). The range of potential refractive error is huge, so it is very helpful to have our patients bring their current <u>glasses</u> in to the office to be measured. These measurements are a starting point for the refraction process. It is also helpful to know the current glasses prescription so that we can advise our patients whether it is "worth it" to update their current spectacles.

refractive error. This is the degree to which you need glasses. Examples of refractive error are <u>nearsightedness</u> or <u>farsightedness</u>. <u>Astigmatism</u> is another refractive error. Your refractive error is obtained with <u>refraction</u>, typically with a phoropter machine in the eye doctor's office.

Refresh. A popular brand of artificial tear (<u>rewetting drop</u>). Refresh comes in different consistencies, including the thicker Refresh PM (a <u>rewetting ointment</u> that can be used at bedtime).

Rescula. This is a new <u>glaucoma</u> drop that has recently "re-entered" the market. This medication is similar to the <u>prostaglandin</u> glaucoma drop latanoprost, but seems to have a slightly different mechanism of action and is not as strong acting. I utilize this drop rarely in my own practice, but it may be good for people who can't tolerate a more powerful prostaglandin and the side effects of beta-blocker drops such as timolol. Rescula may also be a "last ditch" additional drop for people with uncontrolled glaucoma who are already taking every other drop available. It is not clear if Rescula has any added benefit in this setting, however.

Restasis. This is an eye drop with cyclosporine used for treating dry eye. This medication improves both the quantity and quality of the tear film. Unfortunately, it can be expensive (this is getting better), stings going in, and takes a good month before improvement is seen. Also, it doesn't work for everyone. On the other hand, most people with dry eye are desperate for relief so if the drop works, it is worth the hassle. If you develop an eye infection, temporarily stop this medication as it can make viral infections worse. This drop is usually dosed as a single drop twice a day.

Restor lens. This is a multifocal implant using during cataract surgery that can give good distance and near vision without requiring glasses. With cataract surgery, the cloudy lens is removed from the eye and replaced by a plastic "implanted" lens. A new lens is required to see clearly. The standard lens most people opt for is in focus only for far distance, and you still need reading glasses afterward. Newer lenses, like the Restor lens, have a bifocal built into the implant itself and can give good distance AND near vision. This technology is useful for active people who wish to decrease their reliance on spectacles. The technology comes at a price, however, as medical insurance won't pay for the additional cost of this implant. Also, there are some mild visual tradeoffs with multifocal implants such as seeing rings around lights at night.

retina. The retina is the light sensitive structure in the back of the eye that detects images and converts light into signals that our brain can understand. The retina works like "film in a camera." When light enters the eye, it travels through the cornea in the front, through the dark pupil, through the lens/cataract, before striking the retina in the back. The

retina is a pretty remarkable structure because of its high resolution and ability to detect light in very dark situations. The <u>photoreceptors</u> (<u>rods</u> and <u>cones</u>) detect black and white and color light, respectively. The <u>macula</u> is the central area of the retina that is responsible for our central vision. There are more photoreceptors packed in this area to allow high resolution central vision.

retinal detachment. This is when the <u>retina</u> peels off in the back

of the eye, leading to catastrophic vision loss. Because the retina works like film in a camera, it needs to be perfectly smooth and flat to take a good "picture." The retina is plastered smooth against the inner eye like wallpaper. A retinal detachment occurs when the retina begins to peel off (like wallpaper coming off a wall). There are many potential causes for a detachment. Most occur secondary to aging changes in the <u>vitreous</u> jelly that fills the eye. The vitreous is a gel-like fluid that fills the back of the eye. As we age, this jelly liquefies and becomes watery, and then can contract inwards. This contraction is called a <u>vitreous detachment</u> and is almost always a normal and harmless event. However, sometimes the vitreous gel can pull on the retinal surface and create a small tear in the retina. This tear can extend and turn into an actual retinal detachment. There are other causes for detachment, such as traction caused by <u>diabetic retinopathy</u> and even tumors, though these are rare. A detached retina can cause significant vision loss, especially if the <u>macula</u> (the part of the retina responsible for fine central vision) has detached as well. There are many methods for repairing a detachment, depending upon the severity of findings. Lasers can be used to seal a retinal tear. A <u>vitrectomy</u> is often required. This is a surgical procedure where a retina specialist removes the vitreous jelly from the eye in order to remove this as a source of traction. Gas bubbles are sometimes injected to hold the retina in place (a <u>pneumatic retinopexy</u>), and sometimes a silicone buckle (called a <u>scleral buckle</u>) is sewn around the outside of the eye to keep the retina in place.

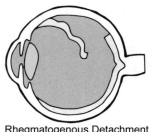 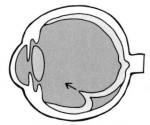 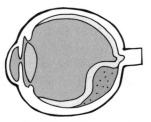

Rhegmatogenous Detachment	Tractional Detachment	Exudative Detachment
(most common)	(seen with diabetic retinopathy)	(rare, associated with tumor)

retina specialist. This is an <u>ophthalmologist</u> (MD) who goes on to sub-specialize in the treatment of <u>retina</u> problems. Retina doctors perform surgeries to correct retinal problems such as <u>retinal detachments</u> and <u>membrane peels</u>. They also treat <u>wet macular degeneration</u>, performing <u>injection</u> procedures and advanced retinal <u>laser</u> procedures. These doctors don't typically perform other eye services such as <u>refraction</u> for glasses, nor do they treat problems like <u>glaucoma</u> or <u>cataracts</u>.

retinitis pigmentosa. A genetic disorder of the <u>retina</u> that causes gradual vision loss. With retinitis pigmentosa (sometimes called RP) the <u>photoreceptors</u> (<u>rods</u> and <u>cones</u> of the retina) or their supporting cells gradually stop working, affecting vision. Some people develop visual loss in infancy while others have problems later in life. Often the rods (the photoreceptors responsible for peripheral and night vision) are involved such that the vision constricts inward making it hard to see in the periphery. Night vision is often severely diminished. There are over 80 different types of retinitis pigmentosa that have been discovered. Some are inherited from family, some occur by recessive mutations that only occur when two parents with the same gene defect have a child. Some kinds of RP are sporadic with no family history at all. There have not been found to be any effective treatments for retinitis pigmentosa, though some retina doctors have tried high levels of vitamin A in the past. There is vigorous ongoing research looking for a cure for this disorder.

retinoscope. This is a hand-held tool the eye doctor uses to estimate refractive error such as nearsightedness, farsightedness, and astigmatism. This tool is challenging to learn and not as accurate as a true phoropter refraction. However, this is often the only method of determining a glasses prescription in a young child or non-verbal patient who can't give feedback while reading an eye chart. The retinoscope can also be used to determine a baseline prescription before refining the glasses prescription using the phoropter.

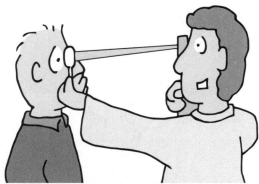

With retinoscopy, a light is shone in the eye and prescription can be estimated by holding up different lenses and examining the red reflections off the retina.

retrobulbar block. This is a more intense way of numbing and paralyzing the eye before difficult eye surgery. Cataract surgery is normally performed under topical anesthesia - simple numbing drops placed on the eye while the patient remains awake. However, if we anticipate that a cataract surgery may take longer than usual (a dense cataract) or may require more manipulation (such as pupil stretching) than a "block" can be considered. With this technique, our patient is temporarily sedated by an anesthesiologist and put completely asleep for about 1-2 minutes. While asleep, the doctor (anesthesiologist or ophthalmologist) injects the retrobulbar numbing agent behind the eyeball itself. This completely numbs the eye and paralyzes the muscles that control eye movement and blinking. This makes the surgery much easier as there is no chance for pain or any unexpected eye movements during the procedure. The downside to a retrobulbar block is that it is more invasive and may require clearance from a primary doctor first. If on blood thinners, these will need to be stopped ahead of time to decrease the chance of bleeding behind the eye from the injection. Finally, the temporary eyelid paralysis means the eye has a harder time closing immediately after surgery and may need to be <u>patched</u> shut overnight to keep the eye from drying out. This is inconvenient and may require a "safety stitch" during the surgery that extends operating time. In our patient population here in Daytona Beach, about one in twenty people require one of these blocks. In other parts of the world where everyone has a terrible, dense cataract (India for example) the majority of surgery is done with a retrobulbar block.

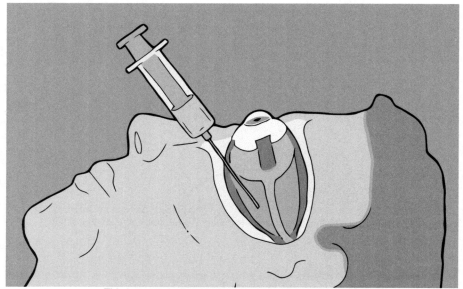

This is a retrobulbar block ... kinda scary looking, huh?

rewetting drops. Also known as artificial tears, these eye drops are designed to comfort and improve lubrication of the eyes. These can be bought over the counter and come with various trade names depending upon the manufacturer. Some popular brands are <u>Soothe</u>, <u>Systane</u>, <u>Blink</u>, and <u>Refresh</u>. Most of these drops contain the same ingredients, differing only by what preservative is used. All eye drops need preservatives (such as <u>BAK</u>) to keep them from getting colonized by bacteria floating in the air and on the eyelashes during use. Unfortunately, these preservatives can be harsh on the ocular surface, which is why we don't recommend using artificial tears more than 4-5 times a day. There are preservative-free eye drops available that come in single use tear-off dispensers. These are great because they can be used frequently without irritating the eye. They can be expensive, however, and they are not as convenient to carry as you can't screw the caps back on. For most people, regular eye drops work fine with the generic drops working just as well as the fancier brand-name drops. If rewetting drops aren't working, then you can also try rewetting gels. These are like rewetting eye drops, but have a thicker consistency and last longer. The downside to the gels is that they make the vision a little blurry when first applied. For people with very dry eyes or exposure issues at night (for example, the eyelids aren't closing all the way when sleeping), rewetting ointments can be effective. These can be bought over the counter, have a consistency similar to Vaseline, and come in squeezable tubes. Ointments make the vision quite blurry so they are best used at bedtime. Popular brands of ointment include Genteel Gel and Refresh PM (the generic alternatives are just as effective).

rewetting gels. These are a type of rewetting drop that have a thicker consistency, similar to shampoo or pancake syrup (but not sticky, obviously). This thickness keeps the drop from evaporating as quickly so that it lasts longer and gives more relief with dry eye. The downside to these gels, however, is that they make the vision a little blurry when first put in. For most people, the additional lubrication is worth the temporary blurriness. Popular brands include Refresh Liquigel and GenTeal gel, but the generics are just as effective. You can find gel drops at the store mixed in with the regular rewetting drops. If the box has "gel" written in its name, you've found the right stuff.

rewetting ointments. These are thick ointments used for extreme dry eye. As rewetting ointments come in tubes they are challenging to put in the eye and the ointment causes significant blurriness to the vision. As such, they are typically reserved for people with extremely dry corneas that aren't adequately covered with traditional rewetting drops and rewetting gels. Some people have eye exposure problems at night. Their eyelids may not close completely while sleeping, which causes a rough or dry spot. The use of oxygen or sleep apnea machines can exacerbate this. In these cases, a rewetting ointment at bedtime will keep the eye lubricated all night long and hopefully make the eyes feel better the next day. To apply, we have our patient pull the lower eyelid down and apply a small amount of ointment (about the size of a grain of rice) to the inside of the eyelid. Then, blink a few times and the vision should get blurry as the ointment spreads over the surface of the eye. It does not take much ointment to lubricate the eye. If you have a difficult time applying an ointment, you may need help from family members. Rewetting ointments are available over the counter without the need for a prescription. They

are located in the same section as the other artificial tears. Popular brands of rewetting ointments include <u>Refresh</u> PM and <u>GenTeal</u> Gel.

RK. This is a surgical procedure where a diamond knife is used to create radial cuts in the <u>cornea</u>. This changes the shape of the ocular surface and can help eliminate <u>nearsightedness</u>. See <u>radial keratotomy</u> for more information on this older refractive surgery.

rod. A type of <u>photoreceptor</u> inside the <u>retina</u> that senses light. Rods are very sensitive and give the eye excellent night vision. Rods can only see in "black and white" in contrast to <u>cones</u>, which are the photoreceptor cells that detect color.

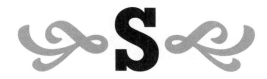

EYE CARTOON

by Tim Root, M.D.

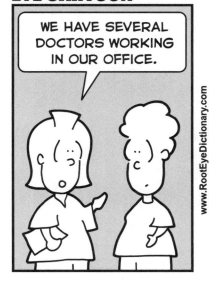

WE HAVE SEVERAL DOCTORS WORKING IN OUR OFFICE.

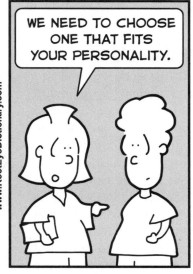

WE NEED TO CHOOSE ONE THAT FITS YOUR PERSONALITY.

www.RootEyeDictionary.com

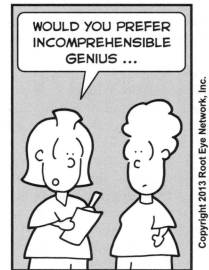

WOULD YOU PREFER INCOMPREHENSIBLE GENIUS ...

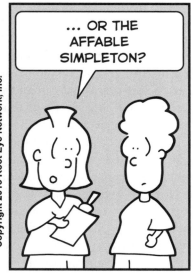

... OR THE AFFABLE SIMPLETON?

sclera. This is the white part of the eye. The sclera is the firm wall of the eye that gives the eye its shape and structure. Made of collagen fiber, the sclera is relatively tough. It is also continuous with the clear cornea in the front of the eye. The sclera is covered by a thin layer of skin called the conjunctiva. This clear skin covers the eyeball and contains small blood vessels you can see in the mirror. When you are looking at the "white" of your eye, you are looking through this conjunctival skin at the scleral wall of the eye itself.

scleral buckle. This is a surgical procedure used to repair a retinal detachment. With this procedure, a silicone band is inserted around the eye and cinched tight, like a belt around a waistline. This decreases traction forces inside the eye which allows the retina to lay back in its normal position. Scleral buckle surgery is widely performed and used 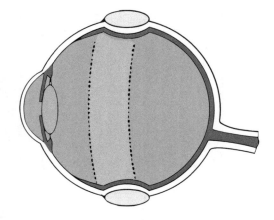 to be the only viable treatment for retinal detachments. Other techniques have arisen such as vitrectomy and pneumatic retinopexy. Every retina specialist has their own surgical preferences and the technique chosen depends upon circumstances and the location of retinal breaks. Some retina surgeons seem to be leaning toward vitrectomy as improvements in retina instrumentation have made vitrectomies fast and less traumatic. There are benefits and risks in all these retinal procedures. One potential problem with a scleral buckle is that the silicone band tends to make the eye physically longer and this can change the overall refractive error of the eye. It's fairly common for the eye to become extremely nearsighted. This can be fixed with a change in glasses prescription, but if the difference between the eyes becomes too great, the glasses won't be comfortable to wear and a contact lens might be required instead. Fortunately, most of these balance issues can be fixed during cataract surgery or with LASIK if they become too bothersome. Less easy to fix is the potential for strabismus, where the buckle makes the eyes slightly out of alignment, causing double vision. Retinal detachments are serious, so these risks are acceptable given the alternative (a blind eye).

second sight. This is the phenomenon where <u>cataract</u> formation seems to make the vision "better" by improving your <u>glasses prescription</u>. A cataract is when the <u>lens</u> inside your eye becomes cloudy. An enlarging cataract usually causes <u>glare</u> problems, but the cataract growth can also change the eye's overall "glasses prescription" as well. For some people, this change is in a bad direction and they require stronger and stronger glasses to see well. For a lucky few, the change is in a "good" direction and actually decreases the reliance on spectacles. The eyes aren't really "improving," it just seems that way. One of the signs that perhaps a cataract is getting worse is when the glasses prescription starts changing rapidly.

shingles. This is a re-outbreak of chicken pox. When people get chickenpox as a child, the viral infection can hit large parts of the body. The body's immune system fights back and eradicates the virus. However, the virus is not completely gone, but usually sits dormant in the base of the nerves in the spine and head. Later in life, as the immune system slows down, the virus can reactivate and run back out the nerve and affect the skin. This outbreak is called "shingles" or "zoster" and it usually affects a single dermatome (strip of skin) in the body. If the fifth cranial nerve of the head (called the trigeminal nerve) is affected, the shingles outbreak can occur on the face. Often the forehead and scalp are involved with painful lesions and swelling of the skin. If the eye is affected this can lead to <u>corneal</u> scaring and long-term vision problems. We usually treat a shingles outbreak with an antiviral medication like <u>Valtrex</u> or <u>acyclovir</u>. If these medications are started within three days of initial symptoms, the medications have been found to limit duration of illness and decrease the chance of long-term sensation/pain problems. It's important to see an eye doctor if there is any eye redness or change in vision as the eye may require treatment as well.

Simbrinza. This is a new combination <u>glaucoma</u> drop combining two separate pressure-lowering medicines - brinzolamide (<u>Azopt</u>) and <u>brimonidine</u> (<u>Alphagan</u>). Combination drugs are useful for decreasing the number of actual drops you must take. The downside, however, is their premium cost is not covered by your prescription drug plan.

Similasan. This is a brand of herbal eye drop therapies. Given the shear number of FDA-approved and scientifically studied eye medicines available, I never bother with this. Someone must be using this, however, since the company is still in business and the product is still on shelves.

sixth nerve palsy. This is a paralysis

of the sixth cranial nerve. This nerve controls a single eye muscle, the abducens muscle, which is responsible for making the eye look to the side. If this muscle stops working the eye turns inward (cross-eyed) and has a hard time moving outwards. Most people complain of a side-by-side horizontal double vision. Like all cranial nerve palsies, there are many potential causes for an abducens palsy. The most common cause is microvascular injury from diabetes or hypertension. You

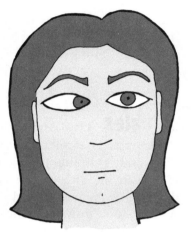

can think of this like a miniature "stroke" to the nerve. Other potential causes are mass lesions (tumors or aneurysms) and high intracranial pressure such as from pseudotumor cerebri. Most sixth nerve palsies are self-limited and improve after a few months. Ophthalmologists used to watch these palsies for spontaneous improvement, but in this day and age of MRI imaging, we tend to image everyone with a new palsy to rule out the dangerous stuff.

slit lamp microscope.

This is a microscope used by an eye doctor to look at the eye. The eye microscope is unique when compared to a traditional microscopes. For one thing, the microscope has been turned on its side so that people can be examined without having to lie down flat. Also, the light-source used can

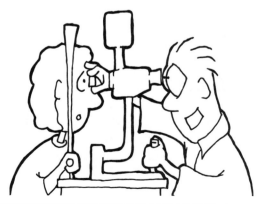

be narrowed to a very narrow beam of light. This light can be angled into the eye to form an illuminated cross-section of the eye ... just like how a CAT scan takes cross-section x-ray slices. The eye is the only place in the body that blood vessels and nerves can be seen without opaque skin blocking the view. With a dilated eye exam, the <u>optic nerve</u> (a direct extension off the brain) can be viewed in great detail. Certain systemic conditions can be observed and diagnosed using the slit lamp microscope. For example, diabetes can cause micro-bleeding in the retina (<u>diabetic retinopathy</u>) and inflammatory conditions like rheumatoid arthritis can cause internal ocular inflammation (<u>uveitis</u>). With the slit-lamp microscope and careful technique, individual white blood cells floating in the eye can be detected.

SLT. This is the abbreviation for Selective Laser Trabeculoplasty - it is a glaucoma laser procedure designed to lower eye pressure in a non-destructive way. Most cases of <u>glaucoma</u> involve microscopic blockage of the <u>trabecular meshwork</u> drain inside the eye. If the internal ocular fluid doesn't drain properly, <u>aqueous</u> fluid pressure builds up and causes gradual damage over time. There are many ways to lower eye pressure. Glaucoma eye drops work to open the drain chemically and you can think of them like "Drano" for the eye. Glaucoma surgery is very effective, but it is also a big production and associated with some morbidity. Fortunately, glaucoma laser therapies have come a long way. <u>ALT</u> was the original laser procedure. With ALT, a "hot" laser was directed at the eye's drain and used to create scars in the <u>trabecular meshwork</u>. These scars helped open drainage tissue to manually get things flowing. This worked really well to lower pressure, but unfortunately the effect is short-lived and tended to wear off after a couple of years. ALT can't be repeated as there is only so much scar tissue the eye can suffer. SLT is a newer laser technology that some people have dubbed as a "cold laser." SLT doesn't create scaring inside the eye, but instead is used to irritate and stimulate the trabecular drainage cells to flow better. The benefit to SLT is that no permanent scars are created and the procedure can be repeated if it wears off. The downside to SLT is that is doesn't work for everyone. We like to think of SLT as an adjunctive therapy to eye drops ... if you are taking a single glaucoma drop, SLT therapy may be able to get you off it. If you are already on glaucoma drops and your eye pressure is creeping up, an SLT treatment may keep you from needing an additional drop or surgery.

The procedure takes about 5 minutes and is painless with little recovery time.

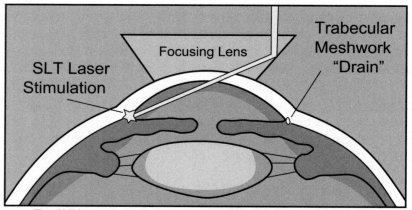

The SLT laser stimulates the drainage cells in the trabecular meshwork, lowering the eye pressure.

Snellen chart. This is the eye chart used by American eye doctors for measuring vision. The letters on this eye chart are calibrated based on distance measurements, comparing your vision to someone with "perfect" eyes. For example, if you have a vision of 20/60 ... this means that the letters you can barely see when standing 20 feet from the chart can be easily seen by a "perfect-eyed person" standing a full 60 feet away from the same chart! In the USA and many European countries, legal driving vision is 20/50 and you are considered <u>legally blind</u> if your *corrected* vision is 20/200 or worse. The Snellen chart is calibrated to be 20 feet from the exam chair you are sitting in ... but few eye doctors have exam rooms this long. To offset this, mirrors are used to obtain the full 20-foot distance.

Soothe. This is a brand name <u>rewetting drops</u> from Bausch & Lomb. Competing brands are <u>Systane</u>, <u>Blink</u>, <u>GenTeal</u>, and <u>Refresh</u>.

squinting. Squinting of the eyes is common, and is commonly done in an attempt to see better. If the eye has <u>refractive error</u> (like <u>nearsightedness</u> or <u>farsightedness</u>) the images entering the eye do not focus well on the <u>retina</u> and look blurry. By squinting and looking through the eyelashes, you can actually see a little clearer. The eyelashes turn the eye into a <u>pinhole</u> camera, which improves depth of focus and improves vision. Squinting is not a good long-term vision solution (obviously), so <u>glasses</u> or <u>contacts</u> are prescribed to improve vision and decrease eye strain. See the entry on <u>pinholes</u> to understand this concept better.

steroid.

Steroids are useful in ophthalmology for treating ocular inflammation. This is particularly useful after <u>cataract surgery</u> and with internal ocular inflammation such as <u>uveitis</u>. Steroids can also be useful for decreasing <u>corneal</u> scarring, such as after a trauma or infection. Care must be used with steroids, however, as they can exacerbate infections - viruses and bacteria love steroids as it "makes them strong." While short term topical steroids are relatively safe, long-term use may cause some problems. Some people are "steroid responders" and their eye pressure tends to go up while on topical eye drops. This pressure change usually takes a few weeks to kick in and goes away after a couple of weeks off the drops. Steroids are also associated with premature cataract formation, though this is more of an issue with oral steroids. Common steroids used by eye doctors are <u>prednisolone</u> acetate (<u>Pred-Forte</u> or <u>Econopred</u>), <u>loteprednol</u> (<u>Lotemax</u> and <u>Alrex</u>) and <u>dexamethasone</u> (usually found in combination drops like <u>Tobradex</u>).

strabismus.

This is a descriptive term used by eye doctors to describe eyes that are in poor alignment with each other. For example, someone with strabismus may be <u>cross-eyed</u>, <u>wall-eyed</u>, or have an eye that drifts upwards. Some people have strabismus that occurs only when tired and others have a problems with <u>double vision</u> only with reading. There are many causes for strabismus, from congenital motor problems to <u>cranial nerve palsies</u>. Strabismus needs to be evaluated by an eye doctor for an appropriate workup. If the alignment problem persists, <u>strabismus surgery</u> is sometimes recommended. <u>Prism</u> glasses are another option, especially for long-standing strabismus in adults.

strabismus surgery.

This is surgery to correct ocular misalignment (<u>strabismus</u>). Most strabismus surgery is performed on toddlers to correct alignment problems such as crossed-eyes. This surgery involves the weakening or strengthening of eye muscles by shortening them or changing their insertion points on the edge of the eye. While most ophthalmologists have trained in performing strabismus surgery, these days the procedure is mostly carried out by pediatric ophthalmologists who have more practice with this type of surgery. Many pediatric ophthalmologists perform adult strabismus surgery as well.

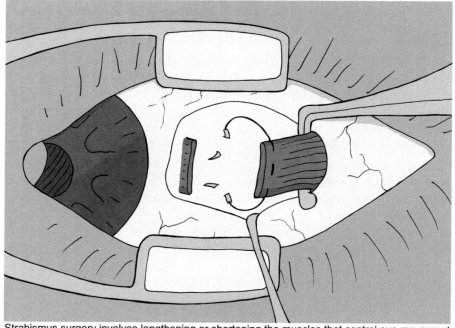

Strabismus surgery involves lengthening or shortening the muscles that control eye movement

stye. A stye is an infection of one of the oil or sweat glands running along the eyelid. Styes are tender to the touch and may form an abscess or pus layer that is visible through the skin as a "white head." The treatment for a stye typically begins with warm compresses and gentle massage. While a "pimple" elsewhere on the body can usually be "popped" or "lanced" with little ill effect, I strongly discourage being too aggressive with the eyelid as the eyeball underneath is a sensitive structure and easily injured. Also, some doctors think that aggressive eyelid squeezing may actually spread infection to adjacent skin and make the stye worse. If warm compresses and gentle massage aren't working, the stye may require topical or oral antibiotics, and even lancing. A stye is a bit different than a chalazion, which is a blockage of the deeper meibomian glands that tends to be painless.

subconjunctival hemorrhage. This is an extremely red eye
that occurs when a blood vessel on the surface of the eye ruptures. The
white part of the eye (the sclera) is covered by a very thin layer of skin
called the conjunctiva. You can see this skin when looking in a mirror, as
red blood vessels course through it and look like "lines" on the eye. If
one of these blood vessels bursts for some reason, such as after a cough
or sneeze, blood will track underneath the conjunctiva and make the eye
look extremely red. It only takes a few drops of blood to make the eye
look bright red and this can look quite alarming in the mirror. A
subconjunctival hemorrhage is almost always harmless, but warrants a
check to make sure there is no bleeding inside the eye (a hyphema or
vitreous hemorrhage) and to make sure the cornea isn't drying out.

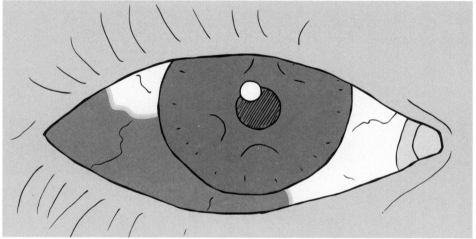

A subconjunctival hemorrhage may look impressive, but is rarely dangerous.

sulfa allergy. Several medicines are sulfa based and can cause
problems for people allergic to sulfa drugs. The main culprits are the
carbonic anhydrase inhibitors used for glaucoma. Examples of these
glaucoma drops include dorzolamide, Trusopt, Azopt, and Cosopt. Also,
the water pill Diamox (acetazolamide) is sometimes used for treating
advanced glaucoma, but is sulfa-based as well. Sulfacetamide is an
antibiotic eye drop (also called Bleph-10) that can also cause sulfa
problems, but I rarely prescribe this, given the plethora of good antibiotic
alternatives.

sulfacetamide sodium 10%. Also known by the trade name Bleph-10, this is an antibiotic eye drop that has gone generic and can be found on the Walmart $4 list. This drug is sulfa-based and not good for those people with sulfa allergy.

Systane. This is a brand name rewetting drop made by Alcon. Competing brands include Soothe, Blink, GenTeal, and Refresh.

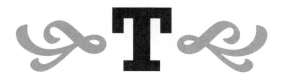

EYE CARTOON

by Tim Root, M.D.

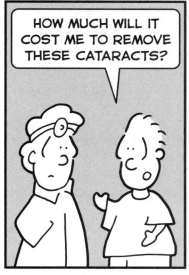

Panel 1: HOW MUCH WILL IT COST ME TO REMOVE THESE CATARACTS?

Panel 2: WE CHARGE ABOUT ONE THOUSAND DOLLARS AN EYE.

Panel 3: ONE THOUSAND DOLLARS FOR A FEW MINUTES WORK? OUTRAGEOUS!

Panel 4: I CAN PERFORM YOUR SURGERY VERY SLOWLY IF THAT WILL HELP.

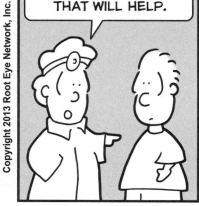

tamsulosin. This is the active ingredient in <u>Flomax</u>, the medication used to help with urinary flow in men with prostate enlargement. Our main concern with this drug is that it can cause <u>floppy iris syndrome</u> during <u>cataract surgery</u>. Floppy iris syndrome is when the iris undulates and moves during a cataract operation and is a potential cause for complications.

tear film. Your tear film is crucial for both good vision and ocular comfort. The tear film is actually composed of three different layers. The innermost layer is made of mucous that helps the tears "stick" to the eye. The middle layer is composed of an aqueous water layer. The surface layer is composed of lipid (oil) that keeps the tear film from evaporating too quickly. This oil is produced by the <u>meibomian glands</u>. For the health of the tear film, both the amount of tears AND the composition of the tear film is important. <u>Rewetting drops</u> usually replace only the middle aqueous layer, while warm compresses can improve the oil production from the meibomian glands. <u>Restasis</u> eye drops may increase the eye's production of tears in certain cases, while <u>punctal plugs</u> keep the tears from draining away too quickly. The tear film is where the majority of light focusing occurs. If this surface has any irregularity to it (from <u>dry eye</u> or excessive tearing) the vision will be severely affected.

tearing. The <u>tear film</u> serves many functions for the eye. Tears lubricate the eye and protect the eye from foreign bodies by washing them away. Tears also help vision by creating a smooth surface for the refraction of light. Too little tears can cause <u>dry eye</u>, where the eyes feel irritated and "tired." Too much and the fluid will collect along the lower eyelid, making the eyes feel weepy and the vision blurry. Tearing can be so bad that the tears overwhelm the nasolacrimal "drain" and roll down the cheek instead (<u>epiphora</u>). Most people with "weepy" eyes actually suffer from dry eye. Their basal tear production is too low, causing intermittent episodes of ocular irritation. When the eyes are irritated, reflexive tearing from the <u>lacrimal gland</u> turns on and floods the eye like a waterfall. This results in periodic episodes of dry eye followed by periods of intense watering. Sometimes, a regularly scheduled regimen of <u>rewetting drops</u> (artificial tears) can help even out this cycle.

temporal arteritis. This is an inflammatory syndrome involving the arteries of the head and neck that can cause serious vision loss. With this condition, the arteries around the head become inflamed. If enough inflammation occurs, an artery can close off and cause sudden neurologic changes. If this happens to the arteries running to the eye, this creates a sudden loss of vision. Symptoms of temporal arteritis include temple pain (especially when brushing hair), jaw claudication (pain when chewing food), unexpected weight loss, night sweats, and general feeling of malaise. Diagnosis is first made by looking for inflammatory markers in the blood (ESR and CRP levels), with a possible biopsy of the temporal artery if a more definitive diagnosis is needed. A biopsy is usually performed by a vascular surgeon only if we feel that the result will change the management of this diagnosis. Treatment is with steroids, usually taken for a prolonged course over many months (sometimes more than a year). Temporal arteritis is considered a disease in the "elderly" and rarely seen under the age of 65. Temporal arteritis is sometimes called "giant cell arteritis" and is related to a systemic condition called polymyalgia rheumatica where similar inflammation occurs throughout the entire body.

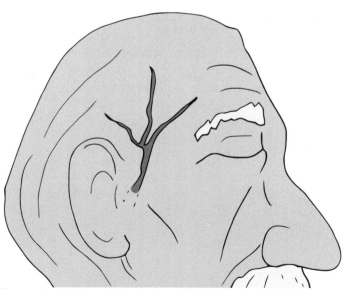

Temporal arteritis is an inflammation of the blood vessels of the head and neck. It can cause serious neurologic problems to the eye.

tetracaine. This is an <u>anesthetic drop</u> used to numb the eye during an eye exam or prior to surgery. Tetracaine works similar to the novacaine that a dentist uses, but can be applied as a simple eye drop. This drop (or a similar drop called <u>proparacaine</u>) is commonly used to anesthetize the <u>cornea</u> prior to checking eye <u>pressure</u> with <u>applanation tonometry</u>. This drop is also used immediately prior to <u>cataract surgery</u> and minor surgical procedures. Tetracaine stings a little going in and will make the eye feel strange for a few minutes. The numbing effect lasts about 10-20 minutes before it begins to wear off. It is important that you not rub your eye while it is numb ... you may be scratching your cornea and cause damage to yourself without realizing it. This drop is never prescribed for home use as repeated applications can actually be toxic to the ocular surface and will keep wounds and <u>corneal abrasions</u> from healing properly.

third nerve palsy. This a paralysis or "stroke" to the third cranial nerve. This nerve is involved with most muscles controlling eye movement. When the nerve is damaged, this causes the eye to turn down and outwards. The third nerve is also involved with controlling <u>pupil</u> size, so a palsy will often make the pupil dilate. Finally, the third nerve helps with eyelid elevation and so a palsy will often cause the eyelid to droop (<u>ptosis</u>). A new third nerve palsy is a potential emergency, especially if the pupil is 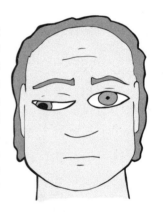 involved, and usually prompts a trip to the hospital to look for aneurysms or mass lesions that might be pushing on the nerve.

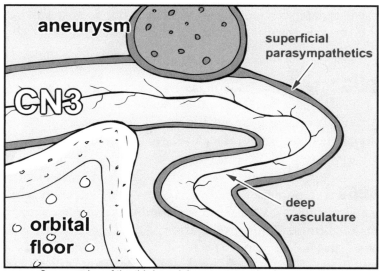

Compression of the third cranial nerve can make the pupil dilate.

thyroid eye disease.
Thyroid dysfunction can cause a number of ocular problems. The most common is dry eye, as the hormonal changes can decrease tear production. Graves disease can stiffen the eye muscles located behind the eyeball and cause fibrous deposits that make the eye muscles swell and expand. This can actually make the eyes protrude forward in a condition called exophthalmos. Thyroid dysfunction can also cause the upper eyelid to retract which can give a person a surprised or wide-eyed appearance. Finally, thyroid muscle dysfunction can cause double vision (diplopia).

timolol.
This is a common beta-blocker eye drop used for treating glaucoma. This drop is usually dosed twice a day. Timolol is an older drop that has been around for a long time, so it is readily available as an inexpensive generic. Punctal occlusion is sometimes recommended to minimize any systemic side effects of timolol (decreased blood pressure and breathing issues in asthmatics).

timolol GFS.
This is a beta-blocker eye drop used for treating glaucoma. The GFS stands for gel forming solution. It is a thicker consistency that allows the drop to be dosed only once a day. An

inexpensive generic version is also available, but is dosed twice a day. Timolol GFS is also available under the trade name Istalol.

Timoptic. This is the trade name for a eye drop containing timolol. This is a beta-blocker medication that lowers eye pressure by decreasing aqueous fluid production inside the eye. I never see this medicine in circulation, as generic timolol is inexpensive and easily obtained.

Tobradex. A popular eye drop used to limit infection and reduce inflammation of the eye. The drop is a combination drug containing two different medicines. Tobramycin is an antibiotic good for treating infections and decreasing bacterial load around the eyelids. Dexamethasone is a steroid used for decreasing inflammation. A competing eye drop with similar action is called Zylet. There is a generic available for Tobradex, but it isn't as cheap as one would expect. We will sometimes prescribe Maxitrol instead - it is very inexpensive, but a little harsh on the eye and not tolerated well by everyone (especially with prolonged use).

Tobradex ST. This is an eye drop used for treating infection and inflammation. It contains both an antibiotic (tobramycin) and a steroid (dexamethasone). This medicine is almost exactly the same as "regular Tobradex," except it is a thicker suspension and designed to work better than the older version (at least, that is what the drug reps keep telling me).

tobramycin. This is an inexpensive antibiotic eye drop with good bacterial coverage. It is readily available and can be found in combination drops such as Tobradex.

tobramycin/dexamethasone. This is a combination drop containing tobramycin (an antibiotic) and dexamethasone (a steroid). Combination drops like this are especially good at treating ocular inflammation caused by blepharitis. In the eye world, we usually refer to this drop by the trade name Tobradex.

Tobrex. This is the trade name for the <u>antibiotic</u> eye drop <u>tobramycin</u>. As tobramycin is available as a very cheap generic, I rarely see "Tobrex" in circulation anymore.

tonometry. This is how we measure the <u>pressure</u> inside the eye. The internal eye pressure is extremely important for the health of the eye. If the pressure is too high, <u>glaucoma</u> damage will occur. If too low, the eye deflates like a water balloon and <u>retinal</u> distortions and <u>macular edema</u> can occur. There are many ways to check the eye pressure, such as the "air puff test," but the one used most often is called the Goldman Applanation Tonometry. This is a small plastic probe that is illuminated with a blue light. As the probe pushes on the eye it flattens a small area of the <u>cornea</u>. The amount of pressure required to flatten the cornea can be used to estimate the internal ocular pressure. This is a relatively accurate device, though <u>corneal thickness</u> can make the readings less so. This <u>applanation tonometry</u> is generally less aggravating then the air puff test. Another tonometry device is called the <u>Tono-Pen</u>. This is a handheld machine that looks like a pen. It is touched to the surface of the eye and works by a similar method. The Tono-Pen is not as accurate as other methods, but is sometimes the only way to accurately measure pressure in a person who is bedridden or who can't get their head into a microscope.

Tono-Pen. A small hand-held electronic machine that is sometimes used to check eye <u>pressure</u>. While not as accurate as other methods, the Tono-Pen is useful for the bedridden and people who can't get up to the microscope for more traditional pressure measurements. To use the Tono-Pen, the eye is numbed with <u>anesthetic drops</u> and the device is gently tapped against the front of the <u>cornea</u>. This doesn't hurt, but feels a little odd. Sterile rubber covers (they look like rubber balloons or miniature condoms) are applied to the Tono-Pen to keep the procedure completely sterile.

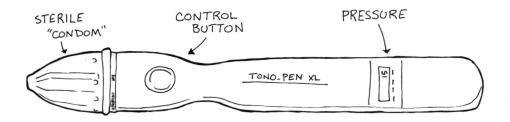

STERILE "CONDOM"   CONTROL BUTTON   PRESSURE

TONO-PEN XL

topography.
In relation to the eye, topography usually refers to corneal topography - this is the measurement of the surface of the cornea. The cornea, the clear window that makes up the front of our eye, works like a fixed-focus lens and actually does the majority of the light focusing in our eye. Irregularities in the corneal surface can have dramatic impact on vision. Corneal topography can be used to measure and map out the corneal surface, similar to mapping out a mountain range in a topographical map. Aberrations like astigmatism can be detected, as can higher-order irregularities such as keratoconus.

toric contacts.
These are contacts designed to help with astigmatism. Normally, the cornea (the clear window that makes up the front of our eye) is perfectly round like a basketball. However, in people with astigmatism, their eye is shaped more like a football ... that is to say, the cornea is steep along one axis and shallower along another. Everyone has a little bit of astigmatism - after all, we are not perfectly round creatures. However, some people have a significant amount of astigmatism and this irregularity can cause some blur to the vision. Astigmatism is relatively easy to fix in glasses. The "football correction" can be ground into a pair of glasses to perfectly offset the eye's football shape. This same process is trickier to pull off with contacts. The football shape can be melted into a plastic contact lens, but contacts have a tendency to spin on the surface of the eye. To counter this, toric contacts are weighted with a thicker bottom so that they line up properly. While this works well, there is no doubt that toric contacts are trickier to fit than a regular contact lens prescription.

toric implants.
These are implants used in cataract surgery designed to counteract the eye's natural astigmatism. Astigmatism is the condition where the eye isn't round, but has an oval shape similar to the

side of a football. This is relatively easy to correct with glasses, as the mirror image of the "football" can be ground into a pair of spectacles and rotated in the glasses frame until the vision is perfected. Astigmatism can now be corrected during cataract surgery using a "toric implant" that has this football correction built in. During cataract surgery, the new toric implant is inserted to replace the old cloudy cataract. The toric implant is then spun until its "football" is lined up to offset the eye's natural astigmatism. While there is no guarantee that a toric lens will keep someone completely "glasses free" after surgery, these implants significantly decrease astigmatism and lessen your dependence on glasses afterward.

Tozal. This is a prescription vitamin used to treat macular degeneration and dry eye. It contains most of the vitamins from the AREDS Study, along with the Omega-3 fatty acids and plant pigments (lutein and zeaxanthin) from the AREDS 2 Study. Tozal also contains taurine, a protein that is commonly found in energy drinks that is "supposed" to increase energy production in the retina. I rarely prescribe this medicine, as good AREDS vitamins (Ocuvite, PreserVision, I-CAPS) are available over the counter without a prescription. I will use it on occasion if your prescription drug coverage is excellent, or I am worried about your getting the proper eye vitamins (such as someone in a nursing home who can't reliably get non-prescription medications).

trabecular meshwork. This is the drain inside the eye where excess aqueous fluid drains and returns back to the bloodstream. This drain is located in a 360-degree ring inside the eye, right where the sclera (the white of the eye) meets the iris (the colored part of the eye). The trabecular meshwork is difficult to see directly, even when using the eye microscope because it is located inside the eye and "around the corner" in the angle of the eye. To help with visualization, a special mirrored-lens can be placed on the surface of the eye. This technique is called gonioscopy and is painless. It is believed that people with chronic open angle glaucoma have something microscopic clogging up the meshwork (like a dirty coffee filter). Other people have narrow angles, such that their drainage angle is tight so that fluid has a hard time reaching the trabecular meshwork to begin with. If this narrow drainage angle closes off entirely, fluid can't drain out of the eye and the ocular pressure shoots up very high. This process is called <u>acute glaucoma</u>, and a person's risk for having a glaucoma attack can be estimated by examining the trabecular meshwork during gonioscopy.

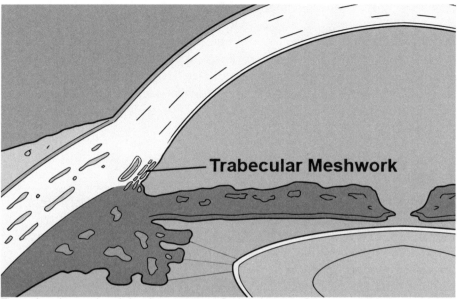

The trabecular meshwork is where aqueous fluid drains out of the eye and is located in the internal "angle" inside the eye. Chronic open-angle glaucoma is likely caused by poor flow through this drain. Acute glaucoma (also known as closed-angle glaucoma) occurs when access to the drain is completely blocked by the iris.

trabeculectomy

. This is a <u>glaucoma</u> surgery, commonly performed to reduce pressure in the eye. Glaucoma occurs because the <u>pressure</u> in the eye is too high. The exact cause for this pressure elevation is unclear, though some people believe that something microscopic is clogging the drain (<u>trabecular meshwork</u>) inside the eye such that <u>aqueous</u> fluid has a hard time leaving the eye. With a trabeculectomy surgery, a new drainage pathway is created so that aqueous fluid from the <u>anterior chamber</u> drains directly to a "pocket" under the <u>conjunctiva</u> skin. This pocket (also called a "bleb") looks like a small blister on the white of the eye under the upper eyelid. Here the aqueous fluid is eventually reabsorbed back into the body. Trabeculectomy is the most common glaucoma surgery performed (more common than <u>tube-shunt</u> surgery). While it is successful at lowering pressure, it does run some long-term risk such as increased chance of internal ocular infection if the bleb ever breaks down. While most <u>ophthalmologists</u> are trained to perform this surgery, we usually leave advanced glaucoma surgeries to glaucoma specialists.

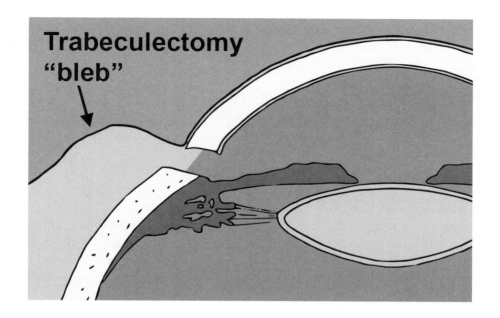

Trabeculectomy "bleb"

trabeculoplasty. This is a <u>glaucoma</u> <u>laser</u> procedure used to improve the flow of <u>aqueous</u> fluid out of the eye. A laser is applied to the <u>trabecular meshwork</u>, which acts as a filter for the fluid leaving the eye. There are two different types of laser therapy used. <u>ALT</u> is a "hot laser" that creates scar spots in the trabecular meshwork that physically open the meshwork to allow drainage. While effective, ALT can only be done once as the eye can only tolerate so much scaring. <u>SLT</u> is a newer laser technology. It is often described as a "cold laser" because it doesn't create the same scaring and can be repeated if necessary.

Travatan. This is a popular <u>glaucoma</u> eye drop medicine. This is a <u>prostaglandin</u> drop and used once daily, usually at bedtime. Competing brands in the same drug class include <u>Lumigan</u> and generic <u>Xalatan</u> (<u>latanoprost</u>).

Travatan Z. This is a <u>glaucoma</u> drop used to lower eye <u>pressure</u>. It is actually the same medicine as regular <u>Travatan</u> (<u>travoprost</u>). However, the manufacturer changed the preservative from <u>BAK</u> to a gentler preservative in an attempt to make the drop less harsh on the corneal surface. Like all <u>prostaglandin</u> glaucoma drops, it is dosed once a day (usually at bedtime).

travoprost. A <u>glaucoma</u> eye drop medication. This is the active ingredient in the eye drops <u>Travatan</u> and <u>Travatan Z</u>. This <u>prostaglandin</u> medication is similar to <u>latanoprost</u> (<u>Xalatan</u>) and thus only needs to be taken once a day.

transitional lenses. These are lenses in <u>glasses</u> that darken when exposed to sunlight. While very effective, they can sometimes take a little while to clear again after you walk inside. Also, transitionals require UV light to change color. Since car windows block UV light (explaining why you don't get sunburned in the car) transitional glasses don't work as well for driving.

triamcinolone. More commonly known as <u>Kenalog</u>, this is a <u>injection</u> <u>steroid</u> used in and around the eye. <u>Retina specialists</u> may inject this medicine into the eye to decrease retinal swelling (<u>macular edema</u>) or to reduce ocular inflammation with recalcitrant <u>uveitis</u>. I occasionally inject this medicine into eyelid lesions, such as <u>chalazions</u>, in order to minimize inflammation and speed up recovery.

trichiasis. This is when <u>eyelashes</u> grow in the wrong direction, rubbing on the surface of the eye and causing irritation. While common, trichiasis is difficult to treat as lashes are thick and the lash follicle hard to destroy. Epilation (plucking) of the eyelashes can be done in the doctors office, though some people with good sight and steady hands are able to pull this off at home with *blunt* tweezers. If persistent, more aggressive surgical correction can be considered.

trifluridine. Also known by the trade name <u>Viroptic</u>, this is an anti-viral drop used primarily to fight <u>herpetic eye disease</u>.

trifocal. These are glasses with three separate zones of focus. The top is set for distance, the middle for intermediate (such as computer distance) while the bottom is optimized for reading. While effective, many people don't like having this many lines on their glasses. For these people, a progressive lens (no line bifocal) may work. Purchasing separate computer glasses may be another option.

tropicamide. This is a dilating drop using during your eye exam. This drop is used in conjunction with phenylephrine to make the pupil dilate to aid in visualizing the lens and retina. Tropicamide is also a short-acting cycloplegia medicine and will make the vision blurry for a couple of hours. This drop is rarely prescribed outside the office, however, as longer acting cycloplegics like atropine and cyclopentolate are more effective in treating eye pain and inflammation. Like all dilating drops, the bottle has a red-colored cap.

Trusopt. Also known as dorzolamide, this is a glaucoma eye drop. This is a carbonic anhydrase inhibitor, which is effective but may be problematic if you have a sulfa allergy. Other medicines in this class of drugs include Azopt (brinzolamide) and the oral medication Diamox. This medicine is also available as the combination drug Cosopt (containing both dorzolamide and timolol).

tube-shunt. This is a surgical procedure performed for severe cases of glaucoma. With glaucoma, the eye pressure is high, which causes gradual death of the optic nerve. There are many ways to lower the eye pressure. Many doctors begin with medicated eye drops. These work to improve the outflow of aqueous fluid from the eye. Other drops decrease the production of aqueous fluid. Laser therapy (such as SLT) can also be performed to improve fluid outflow. If these methods aren't working and visual loss is eminent, a glaucoma surgery can be considered. With a tube-shunt, a small plastic tube is inserted into the anterior chamber in the front of the eye. This tube drains or "shunts" excess aqueous fluid to a pocket under the conjunctiva skin of the eye, up under the eyelid. From here, the vitreous fluid percolates back into the body and is absorbed into the blood stream. This drainage pathway is entirely covered by the conjunctiva skin, so there is no drainage to the outside world. This is important as we don't want to give environmental bacteria an entrance into the eye. Tube-shunt procedures are much more difficult and time consuming than most eye surgeries so are usually reserved for people with advanced or intractable glaucoma.

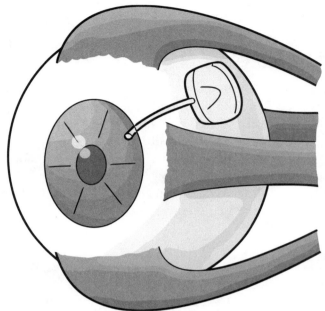

During a tube-shunt surgery, a plastic drainage tube is placed to drain aqueous fluid from behind the eye, thus lowering eye pressure.

twitching eyelid. A twitch or jumping <u>eyelid</u> that tends to come in waves. See <u>eyelid fasciculation</u> for more information.

EYE CARTOON

by Tim Root, M.D.

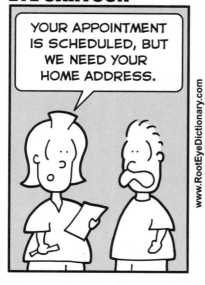

YOUR APPOINTMENT IS SCHEDULED, BUT WE NEED YOUR HOME ADDRESS.

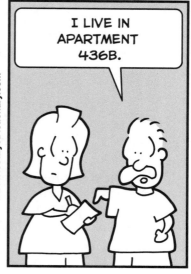

I LIVE IN APARTMENT 436B.

www.RootEyeDictionary.com

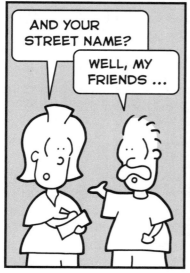

AND YOUR STREET NAME?

WELL, MY FRIENDS ...

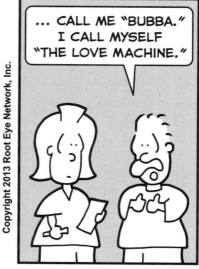

... CALL ME "BUBBA." I CALL MYSELF "THE LOVE MACHINE."

Copyright 2013 Root Eye Network, Inc.

ultrasound. This is the technology where sound waves are bounced off internal organs in order to examine human anatomy. Ultrasound is classically used in the examination of pregnant women, but the technology has some utility in ophthalmology as well. We use ultrasound to measure the length of the eyeball prior to cataract surgery. This measurement is called an A-scan ultrasound. Ultrasound is also useful for examining the eye in cases of vitreous hemorrhage - this is bleeding inside the eye that would otherwise block our view of the retina. We also use ultrasound to examine someone with an extremely dense cataract when our view is blocked by the cloudy lens. The ultrasound technology allows us to check for retinal detachments and other problems inside the eye *before* we subject someone to eye surgery.

uvea. The uvea is an anatomical term used to describe three embryologically related structures in the eye: the iris, ciliary body, and the choroid. The iris is the colored part of the eye and serves as a muscle to control the size of your pupil. The ciliary body is a ring of muscle that sits behind the iris. The ciliary muscle changes the shape of the flexible lens and allows fine visual focusing. The choroid sits under the retina in the back of the eye. The choroid is a bed of blood vessels sitting under the retina that provides oxygen and nourishment to the photoreceptors. The term "uvea" is an anatomical description and is mainly useful in describing the condition uveitis. Uveitis is an inflammation of the uvea structures, and can involve inflammation of the iris, ciliary body, and/or choroid.

uveitis. This is an inflammation inside the eye that involves either the structures in the front of the eye (the iris and ciliary body) or the choroid in the back of the eye. Most people with uveitis have inflammation of the iris (the colored part of the eye). This is called iritis. When the iris is inflamed, it tends to hurt and spasm when subjected to bright lights. This pain is called photophobia. We can detect uveitis when looking inside the eye because we can actually see individual inflammatory cells (white blood cells and macrophages) floating around in the anterior chamber of the eye. The number of these cells visible correlates with the severity of inflammation. If the inflammation is bad enough, the pupil can become irregularly shaped from iris synechiae formation. There are many causes for an episode of uveitis, though at least half of them occur idiopathically with no known cause. Inflammatory conditions like rheumatoid arthritis and sarcoidosis may cause uveitis. People who have HLA-B27 positive conditions like ankylosing spondylitis and inflammatory bowel disease are also prone to uveitis. Viral infections from <u>zoster</u> (<u>shingles</u>) can cause uveitis, especially with repeat outbreaks. Rare infections such as Lyme disease, syphilis, and tuberculosis can all cause uveitis as well (though we seldom see these infections in this area). Treatment is primarily with <u>steroid</u> eye drops (to cool down the inflammation) and a dilating <u>cycloplegia</u> drop (for pain control and to avoid synechiae formation). The first time a person has uveitis, no further workup is usually indicated. However, recurrent or severe bouts may instigate additional testing and consultation with a rheumatologist to look for underlying pro-inflammatory conditions.

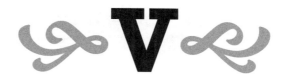

EYE CARTOON

by Tim Root, M.D.

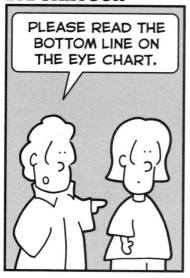

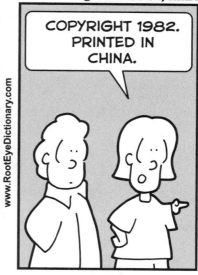

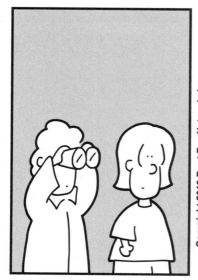

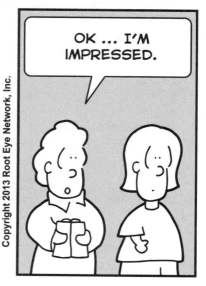

www.RootEyeDictionary.com

Copyright 2013 Root Eye Network, Inc.

valacyclovir. This is an antiviral pill, used in ophthalmology for cases of <u>herpetic eye disease</u> or with <u>shingles</u> (zoster) outbreaks. This medicine is usually referred to as the trade name <u>Valtrex</u>.

Valtrex. This is the trade name for <u>valacyclovir</u>, an antiviral pill used in cases of viral eye infection (such as <u>herpetic eye disease</u> or a <u>shingles</u> infection). It is longer lasting than the alternative <u>acyclovir</u>, so it doesn't have to be taken as frequently. Valtrex may be slightly more powerful than acyclovir as well.

vancomycin. This is a "hard core" IV <u>antibiotic</u> that is traditionally used for hospitalized patients with MRSA infections. We use vancomycin eye drops when treating bad <u>corneal ulcers</u>. This medicine is not available in eye drop form and must be specially created by a compounding pharmacy as a <u>fortified antibiotic</u> drop.

Varilux. This is a high quality progressive lens used in no-line <u>bifocals</u>. <u>Progressive lenses</u> are a type of no-line bifocal that gets stronger the further down the <u>glasses</u> you look. Many people like progressive lenses because they can "dial in" the amount of bifocal they need by tilting their head. Other people find progressives uncomfortable, however, because of the distortion in their lower vision. The Varilux brand of progressive lenses are of a higher quality and seem to be better tolerated with less distortion.

VEGF. This stands for Vascular Endothelial Growth Factor. VEGF is a hormone released from the <u>retinal</u> cells when they become hungry for oxygen. This hormone is meant to stimulate the formation of new blood vessels. The most common causes of VEGF over production are from <u>diabetic retinopathy</u> or a <u>central retinal vein occlusion</u>. When VEGF is released, new blood vessels form to supply the oxygen demand. This process is called <u>neovascularization</u>. Unfortunately, these new blood vessels are abnormal and have a tendency to bleed, scar, and contract, leading to serious visual consequences. <u>Anti-VEGF</u> medications are the hottest topic in ophthalmology these days because these medications can be injected into the eye to fight off these bad vessels. Anti-VEGF medications also decrease capillary leakage, which has made them a good treatment for <u>wet macular degeneration</u> as well. <u>Avastin</u> is the first of the anti-VEGF drugs. Since its advent, there have been newer drug variations that may be more specific for the eye such as <u>Lucentis</u> and <u>Eylea</u>. All of these medications are injected directly into the eye so that they can target the retina directly with less systemic side effects.

vertex distance
. This is the distance measured from the eye surface (the <u>cornea</u>) to the back of a <u>glasses</u> lens. This distance is different for everyone, but on average is about 1.4 centimeters. This measurement can be important when choosing and fitting glasses frames (especially with strong glasses prescriptions). Vertex distance is also important when converting a <u>glasses prescription</u> to a <u>contact</u> lens prescription.

Vigamox
. This is a powerful <u>fluoroquinolone</u> <u>antibiotic</u> containing <u>moxifloxacin</u>. This is an excellent antibiotic for treating corneal infections, especially in <u>contact</u> lens wearers. Alternative brands like <u>Moxeza</u> have come out with the same active ingredient. Similar antibiotic medications include <u>Zymaxid</u> (<u>gatifloxacin</u>) and <u>Besivance</u> (besifloxacin).

viral conjunctivitis
. Also known as "pink eye," this is a viral infection in the eye that makes the <u>conjunctiva</u> red and irritated. The conjunctiva is the thin layer of skin that covers the white of your eye. This skin layer is extremely thin, but you can see it when looking in the mirror as blood vessels course through the skin. When you get an infection of this delicate skin layer, the blood vessels dilate and the eye appears to be "pink." In adults, the majority of eye infections (<u>conjunctivitis</u>) are from viral sources - it's like getting the flu, but instead of getting head or chest congestion, the eye is involved. Just as with the flu, there is no good treatment for viral infections other than letting the infection run its course. Viral conjunctivitis is highly contagious. If you have it, wash your hands frequently and don't share towels or makeup. It may take up to two weeks for the infection to clear and the conjunctivitis may jump to the other eye before the end. If there are any visual changes, the eye needs to be rechecked to make sure there is no corneal involvement (i.e., <u>corneal ulcer</u> formation).

Viroptic. This is an eye drop containing <u>trifluridine</u> that is used to fight viral infections of the eye, such as in <u>herpetic eye disease</u>. While effective, the drop can be a little harsh on the ocular surface with prolonged use. Sadly, there aren't many antiviral alternatives available in this country. <u>Zirgan</u> is a new antiviral ointment that may be better tolerated as it requires less frequent dosing.

Visine. Visine is a brand of over-the-counter eye drops. The original formula contained the drug tetrahydrozoline, a stimulant that makes the blood vessels on the surface of the <u>conjunctiva</u> constrict and shrink. This makes the eyes look whiter and thus it "gets the red out." This effect is short-lived and many people have a rebound effect where the eye turns redder after the drug wears off. Overall, Visine doesn't fix anything and may not be healthy as it decreases blood supply to the irritated tissues. Johnson & Johnson has expanded the Visine brand name to include an entire line of rewetting and allergy drops, so read the label to see what you're actually buying.

vision. The most important component of an eye exam is the measurement of the actual quality of the central vision. We measure this by having you read an eye chart (the <u>Snellen chart</u>) and tweaking the vision by having you look through the <u>phoropter</u> (the machine with all the lenses inside used for checking your prescription). Some patient's vision is so bad that we can't measure and document vision using an eye chart. In these cases we measure other things, like the ability to count fingers and see hand movement. If the vision is really bad, we measure the detection of light. Most of these measurements require feedback from our patients, which makes visual acuity hard to check in young children or non-verbal patients. In these cases we estimate vision by seeing if the eye tracks objects and blinks to bright lights.

visual field. This is a test to measure your peripheral vision. There are many ways to check side vision, but when we say we're going to get a "visual field" we are usually talking about the Humphrey Visual Field. This is a computer-controlled machine that maps out peripheral vision in an objective and precise manner. You wear an eye patch over one eye and sit forward in a bowl of light. While you stare straight ahead at a fixed point, the computer shines a spot of light in various places in your peripheral vision. Every time you see the light, you click the buzzer and the computer maps this data for us. Visual fields are very useful for detecting vision loss in patients with glaucoma. Because a third of the brain is devoted to the visual pathway (and processing of visual images), neurologic problems can be detected and localized with a visual field as well.

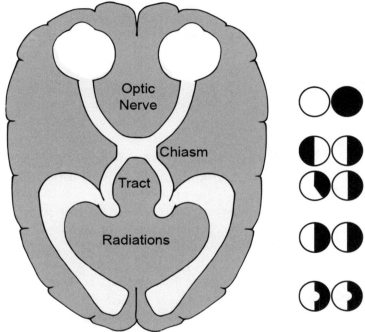

Damage in the brain can often be localized by the visual field pattern measured

vitamins. There has been much research on the effect of vitamins on the eye. Vitamin A in particular seems to be important to the health of the rods and cones as this vitamin is key to the conversion of light images into an electrical signal that can be interpreted by our brain. One of the treatments attempted for people with retinitis pigmentosa (a derangement of the photoreceptors) is high doses of Vitamin A. Other vitamins have been studied in relation to macular degeneration. The AREDS Study found that a combination of Vitamin A (beta-carotene), C, and E (along with the minerals zinc and copper) seemed to slow the progression of vision loss in macular degeneration. See the AREDS Study and AREDS 2 Study for more information on this topic.

vitrectomy. This is a surgery to remove the <u>vitreous</u> fluid from the back of the eye and replace it with saline water. This procedure is performed by a <u>retinal specialist</u> and is commonly performed to help repair <u>retinal detachments</u>. Vitrectomy is also used to remove blood from a <u>vitreous hemorrhage</u> and as part of <u>membrane peel</u> surgery for <u>epiretinal membranes</u> and <u>macular holes</u>. This surgery used to take many hours to perform, but with modern techniques and shrinking instrumentation, it is becoming faster and less traumatic.

vitreous. This is the fluid that fills the back of the eye. The eye is mostly a hollow structure. The large back chamber is filled with vitreous humor, which is a fluid that has the consistency of Jell-O. In fact, if you were to "theoretically" open up a young person's eye and remove the contents, the vitreous would come out as a single glob of clear "goop." As we get older, the vitreous begins to liquefy, with pockets of saline water forming inside the gel. At some point in our life, the mixture gets so watery that the remaining gel will contract inwards upon itself and cause <u>flashes</u>, <u>floaters</u>, and sometimes a <u>retinal detachment</u>. This contraction event is common and called a <u>vitreous detachment</u>.

vitreous detachment. A common cause for <u>flashes</u> and <u>floaters</u>, a vitreous detachment is when the "gel" in the back of the eye contracts inwards upon itself. Let me explain. The eye is mostly a hollow structure. In many ways, the eye is like a water balloon sitting inside your eye socket. The eye is not filled with water, however, but is filled with a clear fluid called the <u>vitreous</u> jelly. This jelly has the consistency very much like Jell-O. In childhood, the vitreous gel is firm and well-formed, but as we get older the gel gets "runny" and "watery." Little pockets of saline water form inside the gel, and while this sounds bad, it really isn't a problem. Both the gel and the water are clear and we can see through them just fine. At some point in our life the vitreous gel can become so watery that one day, without warning, the remaining vitreous gel can suddenly collapse inward upon itself. This causes flashing lights and floaters. If you want to use a metaphor, think of the eyeball like a Tupperware bowl filled to the brim with Jell-O. Now, imagine what would happen if you put that bowl of Jell-O on your kitchen counter and then you went on vacation for several months. With time, the Jell-O will evaporate and dehydrate until it collapses and falls in upon itself like a big "blob" in the middle of the bowl. A similar process happens inside the eye. The vitreous gel peels off the <u>retina</u> inside the eye. The retina detects light, so that as the gel peels off it, many people will see a flash of light like a lightning bolt in their peripheral vision. In addition, many people complain of a new, large floater in their vision. This occurs when a little bit of cellular debris pulls off the <u>optic nerve</u> as the gel peels away from it. This little piece of junk is now floating inside the eye, hovering at the gel-water interface, casting shadows inside the eye that you can see as the gel wobbles around. In rare cases, the vitreous gel can actually rip a small hole in the retina itself. This is bad, because a retinal hole can extend and turn into a full-on <u>retinal detachment</u> with loss of vision. Anyone with new symptoms of flashing lights or new floaters needs a dilated eye exam to look for these retinal tears. If the initial retinal examination shows a healthy retina, I usually have my patients return in a few weeks for a recheck to make sure nothing new has formed. The flashing lights and floaters will diminish with time, though the floater can sometimes take a long time (months or years) to disappear (and sometimes it never does entirely). There is no safe way to make these floaters go away short of a <u>vitrectomy</u> surgery (not recommended).

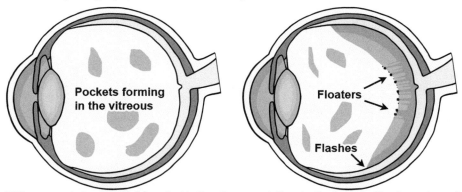

With age, pockets of "water" form inside the vitreous gel. Eventually, the gel will collapse inward and "detach" from the surface of the retina. We see flashing lights from retinal irritation and floaters from new debris hovering over the retina surface.

vitreous hemorrhage.
This is the term used to describe blood inside the eye, specifically blood in the <u>vitreous</u> fluid that fills the back of the eye. Symptoms of a vitreous hemorrhage include <u>floaters</u> and a "dark cloud" that seems to obscure vision. The most common cause for an internal ocular bleed is <u>neovascularization,</u> abnormal blood vessels inside the eye (usually from diabetes) that bleed easily. Other causes of a

hemorrhage are from trauma (obviously) or even a <u>retinal detachment</u>. If the hemorrhage is mild, the blood will usually break down and reabsorb by itself. In these cases, I recommend my patients sleep on their side or with the head of the bed elevated (so that blood doesn't settle in the middle of the vision). Also, you should avoid heavy lifting and blood thinners (if possible) to minimize the chance of rebleeding. Extensive vitreous hemorrhages are more difficult to live with and may require a <u>vitrectomy</u> to restore useful vision in a more timely manner. The underlying cause of any hemorrhage needs to be determined, and if the bleeding IS from something like <u>diabetic retinopathy</u>, treatment with a <u>PRP</u> laser may be the next step.

Voltaren. This is an <u>NSAID</u> eye drop designed to decrease inflammation in the eye (similar to Motrin or Advil). The active ingredient <u>diclofenac</u> is now available as a generic. While effective, this drop can be a little harsh on the ocular surface for some people. Other similar drops include <u>Nevanac</u> (<u>nepafenac</u>) and <u>Bromday</u> (<u>bromfenac</u>).

W

EYE CARTOON   by Tim Root, M.D.

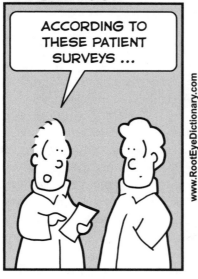

ACCORDING TO THESE PATIENT SURVEYS ...

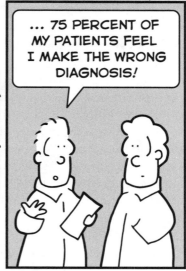

... 75 PERCENT OF MY PATIENTS FEEL I MAKE THE WRONG DIAGNOSIS!

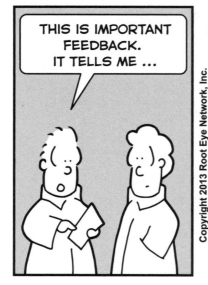

THIS IS IMPORTANT FEEDBACK. IT TELLS ME ...

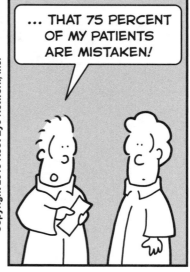

... THAT 75 PERCENT OF MY PATIENTS ARE MISTAKEN!

www.RootEyeDictionary.com

Copyright 2013 Root Eye Network, Inc.

wall-eyed. A simple way to describe eyes that turn outward. This term isn't really used in medicine, but is very descriptive. We would usually describe a wall-eyed person as having an <u>exotropia</u>. The opposite would be <u>cross-eyed</u> (<u>esotropia</u>). Ocular alignment problems like this are called <u>strabismus</u>. New cases of strabismus need to be evaluated by an eye doctor.

wall fracture. In the world of medicine, a "wall fracture" generally implies the breakage of one of the bones that make up the eye socket. The eye socket (also known as the orbit) is constructed from seven different bones inside the skull. Many of these bones are thin and prone to cracking after blunt trauma to the eye. The floor of the orbit is most likely to fracture with injury, and the contents of the eye socket (mainly fat and eye muscle) can herniate down through this fracture into the sinus cavity underneath. While this sounds pretty awful, this crumple zone is actually designed to protect the eye from compressive injuries. In many ways, you can compare our skull's sinuses to the bumpers or airbags in a car. These structures are designed to break in order to protect the important passengers (in this case, the eye and brain). Fortunately, small bone fractures heal on their own without long-term problems. Rarely, a large wall fracture will cause the eye to look sunken inward (enophthalmos) or one of the eye muscles will get caught in the fractured bone. This may require surgical repair. Orbital wall repairs are usually done with an oculoplastics specialist or ENT doctor in the operating room.

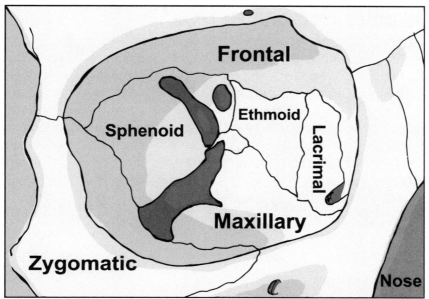

The eye socket (orbit) is made from seven different bones. The maxillary bone that makes up the "floor" of the orbit is the bone most likely to fracture in the event of a blunt trauma to the eye. This can be a problem if any eye muscles get stuck in the fracture. This is sometimes described as a "trap door" effect.

warm compresses. A warm compress can be used to treat many eye conditions. For example, warm compresses can be used with <u>dry eye</u> to improve <u>tear</u> flow. Warmth is also useful in cases of <u>blepharitis</u> to increase the flow of oil from the <u>meibomian glands</u>. Warm compresses are usually recommended in cases of <u>chalazion</u> or <u>styes</u> as they help drain them faster and heat-induced dilation of blood vessels can help oral antibiotics target the involved skin. There are many ways to apply a warm compress. Most people find it easiest to fill a bowl with warm water, dip a washcloth in the water, and apply the damp cloth to the closed eyes. The cloth cools quickly so the process can repeated several times. Other people like to use warm packs with the eyes, though care must be used to not burn the sensitive eyelids.

wet macular degeneration. This is the more serious form of macular degeneration associated with acute swelling in the retina. Macular degeneration can be thought of as a premature aging of the macula, the part of the retina responsible for good central vision. Most people have dry macular degeneration, which is a slow and progressive loss of vision. A certain percentage of these people develop "wet" degeneration where abnormal blood vessels under the retina begin to bleed suddenly. This bleeding causes sudden and severe vision loss as the retina swells with macular edema. Fortunately, the treatment for wet degeneration has improved with the development of anti-VEGF injections such as Avastin and Lucentis.

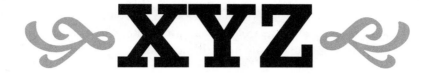

EYE CARTOON

by Tim Root, M.D.

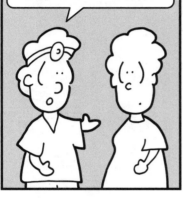

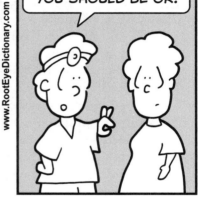

www.RootEyeDictionary.com

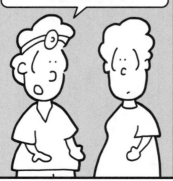

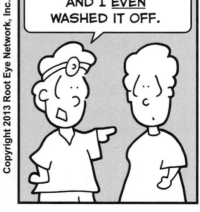

Copyright 2013 Root Eye Network, Inc.

Xalatan. This is a popular <u>glaucoma</u> eye drop. Xalatan was the first <u>prostaglandin</u> drop available and is considered by many doctors the best initial treatment for glaucoma given its action and easy dosing. This drop is taken only once a day, usually at bedtime. This drug is now available as the generic drop <u>latanoprost</u>. Alternative drops in the same drug class include <u>Travatan</u>, <u>Lumigan</u>, and preservative-free <u>Zioptan</u>.

YAG capsulotomy.

This is a <u>laser</u> procedure used to treat "<u>after cataracts</u>." With <u>cataract surgery</u>, the natural <u>lens</u> is removed from the eye and replaced with a plastic lens (see <u>implant</u>). While very successful, some people will form a haze or cloudy membrane on the back of their implant. These "after cataracts" occur months or years after surgery and are not a complication or problem ... but they can cause blurry vision similar to the original cataract. Fortunately, the opacity is easy to remove using a "YAG laser." During the procedure, you sit forward into a laser microscope while I create a hole through the cloudy membrane using tiny laser pulses. This is a painless procedure and takes about 30 seconds to complete. Afterwards, your vision is blurry from the dilating drops but the vision improves rapidly. While this procedure is easy and relatively safe, we recheck your eye in a few weeks to insure no retinal problems have developed. This also gives us a chance to recheck your eye glasses prescription. Once the "after cataract" is gone, it doesn't come back so you don't have to have this procedure repeated ever again.

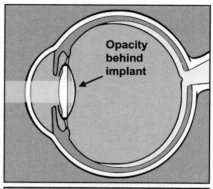

Opacity behind implant

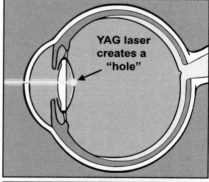

YAG laser creates a "hole"

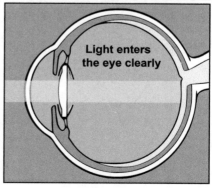

Light enters the eye clearly

Zaditor. This is a popular over-the-counter allergy eye drop. It is useful for ocular itching and swelling and is, in my opinion, one of the best allergy drops available without a prescription. The active ingredient is ketotifen, which is also found in the allergy drop Alaway. This medicine lasts about 12 hours so is usually dosed twice a day.

zeaxanthin. This is a natural pigment produced by plants and absorbed by animals. This pigment is what gives corn its yellow color. This pigment, along with lutein, has been studied as part of the AREDS 2 Study and found to help slow down the progression of macular degeneration. Both these pigments are found in high concentrations inside the retina.

Zioptan. This is a preservative-free prostaglandin drop used for glaucoma. It works similar to Xalatan but comes in individual single-dose dispensers. The active ingredient is tafluprost. This medicine is best used for people with sensitive eyes or who are consistently running out of their regular prostaglandin drop.

Zirgan. An antiviral eye ointment containing ganciclovir. This drug is very effective for the treatment of herpetic eye disease. This is a newer medication and can sometimes take pharmacies a few days to fill. Unfortunately, there aren't many antiviral alternatives available in the US (just Viroptic drops).

zonules. These are string-like attachments that suspend the lens inside your eye. The zonules run around the periphery of the lens/cataract like trampoline springs and attach to the ciliary body muscle. Muscle contraction of the ciliary body changes the tension on the zonules, and this controls the lens shape to help with visual focus. Certain conditions like Marfan syndrome can cause a weakness to the zonules and make the eye prone to lens dislocations as the zonules break. Pseudoexfoliation syndrome can cause the zonules to become brittle and delicate, making cataract surgery challenging because of the resulting zonular weakness.

zoster. This is the term used for chicken pox (varicella zoster) in adults. While rarely a vision problem in childhood, chicken pox can reactivate in adulthood and cause an attack of <u>shingles</u> that can affect the eye.

Zylet. This is a combination drop containing <u>loteprednol</u> (a <u>steroid</u>) and <u>tobramycin</u> (an <u>antibiotic</u>). This combination is especially useful for mild infections and <u>blepharitis</u> (chronic eyelid inflammation). Comparable drops include <u>Tobradex</u> and generic <u>Maxitrol</u>.

Zymar. This is the trade name for the antibiotic eye drop <u>gatifloxacin</u>. This is a powerful <u>antibiotic</u> used for eye infections, <u>corneal ulcers</u>, and after eye surgery. This drug comes in a concentration of 0.3% and is now being supplanted by the medication <u>Zymaxid</u>, which contains the same drug but at a higher concentration. Comparable <u>fluoroquinolone</u> antibiotics in the same drug class include <u>Vigamox</u> and <u>Besivance</u>.

Zymaxid. This is the trade name for <u>gatifloxacin</u> 0.5%. This is the same medicine in <u>Zymar</u> but reformulated with a higher drug concentration. This <u>fluoroquinolone</u> <u>antibiotic</u> is used primarily with bad eye infections and as prophylactic treatment before and after <u>cataract surgery</u>.

⪻Extra⪼

www.RootEyeDictionary.com

Copyright 2013 Root Eye Network, Inc.

EYE CARTOON

by Tim Root, M.D.

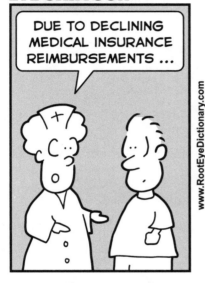

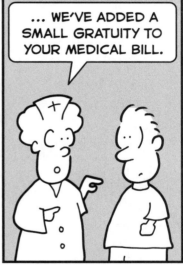

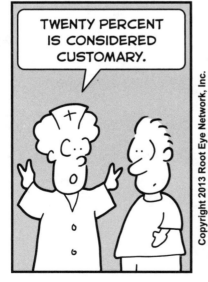

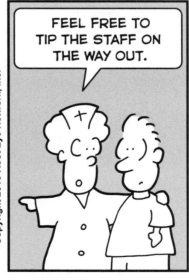

Abbreviations

I suspect that most people who read this book have no interest in eye abbreviations. However, this dictionary (especially the online version) has been popular with students, technicians, and medical coders ... and so I feel compelled to include a list of the most common "abbreviations" used in the field.

A or Acc	accommodation
AC	anterior chamber
AC/A	accommodative convergence/accommodation ratio
ACIOL	anterior chamber intraocular lens
ALT	argon laser trabeculoplasty
APD	afferent pupil defect
ARMD	age-related macular degeneration
ASC	anterior subcapsular cataract
BC	base curve
BD	base down (prism)
BI	base in (prism)
BID	twice a day
BLP	bare light perception
BTL	blink to light
BO	base out (prism)
BRAO	branch retinal artery occlusion
BRVO	branch retinal vein occlusion
BU	base up (prism)
CACG	chronic angle closure glaucoma
CE	cataract extraction
CF	confrontational fields or count fingers

CL	....	clear, contact lens
CLARE	....	contact lens associated red eye
CRAO	....	central retinal artery occlusion
CRVO	....	central retinal vein occlusion
CS	....	conjunctiva and sclera
CSME	....	clinically significant macular edema
CSR	....	central serous retinopathy
D	....	diopter
DFE	....	dilated fundus exam
DLK	....	diffuse lamellar keratitis
DQ	....	deep and quite
DR	....	diabetic retinopathy
E	....	esophoria
E'	....	esophoria at near
EOG	....	electro-oculogram
EOM	....	extraocular movements
ERG	....	electroretinogram
ERM	....	epiretinal membrane
ET	....	esotropia
E(T)	....	intermittent esotropia
EXT	....	extremities
FA	....	fluorescein angiography
FC	....	finger counting
FOL	....	follicles
F/U	....	followup
GL(S)	....	glaucoma suspect
HE	....	hard exudates
HM	....	hand movement
HSV	....	herpes simplex virus
HST	....	horse shoe tear

HT	....	hypertropia
I	....	iris
IMHO	....	in my humble opinion
IOL	....	intraocular lens
IOOA	....	inferior oblique overaction
IOP	....	intraocular pressure
J1,J2	....	Jaeger (near vision scale J1+=20/20)
K	....	cornea
KCN	....	keratoconus
KPs	....	keratic precipitates
L	....	lens
LASIK	....	laser in situ keratomileusis
LOL	....	laugh out loud
LP	....	light perception
LPI	....	laser peripheral iridotomy
LL	....	lids and lacrimation
LLL	....	left lower lid
LUL	....	left upper lid
MA	....	microaneurysms
MP	....	membrane peel
NI	....	no improvement
NLP	....	no light perception
NPDR	....	non-proliferative diabetic retinopathy
NSC	....	nuclear sclerotic cataract
NV	....	neovascularization
NVA	....	neovascularization of the angle
NVD	....	neovascularization of the disk
NVE	....	neovascularization elsewhere
NVG	....	neovascularization glaucoma
NVI	....	neovascularization of iris

NFL	....	nerve fiber layer
OD	....	oculus dexter (the right eye)
ONH	....	optic nerve head
OS	....	oculus sinister (the left eye)
OU	....	oculus uterque (both eyes)
P	....	pupils
Pap	....	papillae
PAS	....	peripheral anterior synechiae
PCIOL	....	posterior chamber intraocular lens
PCO	....	posterior capsular opacification
PD	....	pupillary distance
PDR	....	proliferative diabetic retinopathy
PED	....	pigment epithelial detachment
PED	....	persistent epithelial defect
PEE	....	punctate epithelial erosion
PEK	....	punctate epithelial keratopathy
PERRLA	....	pupils equally round and reactive to light and accommodation
PH	....	pinhole
PHNI	....	pinhole no improvement
PHPV	....	persistent hyperplastic primary vitreous
PI	....	peripheral iridotomy
PK	....	Penetrating keratoplasty (corneal xpl)
POAG	....	primary open angle glaucoma
PPV	....	pars plana vitrectomy
PRP	....	panretinal photocoagulation
PSC	....	posterior subcapsular cataract
PTC	....	pseudotumor cerebri
PVD	....	posterior vitreous detachment

PVR	....	proliferative vitreoretinopathy
PXS/PXF	....	pseudoexfoliation syndrome
QAM	....	morning
QD	....	once a day
QHS	....	nighttime or bedtime
QID	....	four times a day
RAPD	....	relative afferent papillary defect
RD	....	retinal detachment
ROFL	....	roll on floor laughing
RLL	....	right lower lid
ROP	....	retinopathy of prematurity
RP	....	retinitis pigmentosa
RPE	....	retinal pigment epithelium
RUL	....	right upper lid
Rx	....	prescription
Sc	....	sans correction (no glasses)
SCH	....	subconjunctival hemorrhage
SLE	....	slit-lamp exam
SLK	....	superior limbic keratoconjunctivitis
SOOA	....	superior oblique overaction
SPK	....	superficial punctate keratopathy
SRF	....	subretinal fluid
Sph	....	spherical lens
T	....	pressure
Tap	....	pressure (via applanation)
TID	....	three times a day
Tono	....	pressure (via Tono-Pen)
V or Va	....	vision or visual acuity
Vcc	....	vision (with correction)
VEP	....	visual evoked potential

Vsc	....	vision (sans correction)
VH	....	vitreous hemorrhage
Vit	....	vitreous
VMT	....	vitreo macular traction
W&Q	....	white and quite
WNL	....	within normal limits
XOXO	....	hugs and kisses
XT	....	exotropia
X(T)	....	intermittent exotropia

Doctor Root's Publications

The fun doesn't have to stop here! If you want to learn more about the eye, check out some of Dr. Root's other publications:

1. OphthoBook:

A Student's Introduction to the Eye

Available on Amazon and bookstores
www.OphthoBook.com

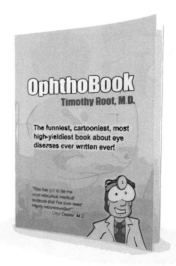

OphthoBook is a medical textbook Dr. Root wrote during his surgical training. This book is available in bookstores and online through retailers such as Amazon. The book is used worldwide by medical students and has been translated into several languages. The OphthoBook website (www.ophthobook.com) brings in 60,000 unique visitors every month. For a preview, we've included the prologue here:

OphthoBook: An Unconventional Path

By Timothy Root, M.D.

There are traditional ways to write a book. For most people, this involves picking a topic, preparing a rough draft, and submitting a manuscript to publishers around the country. If you're lucky, you'll land a small contract. If you're extremely lucky, Oprah will read your novel and a succession of movies might occur, possibly starring Tom Hanks.

Medical books are a little different. The audience for textbooks is small, so medical books are published in small batches and sold at premium prices. Basic macro-economics tell us that this is the way to maximize profit. Supply and demand, baby!

But what if your goal ISN'T to make tons of money? What if your goal is to reach as many people in the world as possible and teach them about eye disease? That was the dilemma I faced as I finished the original manuscript for OphthoBook. The last thing I wanted was for a publisher to buy the rights to my work, sell a few hundred copies at inflated cost, and then let it go out of print. These "literary graveyards" are every author's nightmare.

I took a different path – one that was both easier and yet more challenging. I published this book on the internet as a free download. Instead of contracts, editors, and book signings, I learned website design, search engine optimization, and viral marketing!

Fortunately, this unconventional tactic worked. Over the past four years, approximately 300,000 people have visited my little book's website, watched my video lectures, and downloaded the chapter files.

This is an impact of magnitude greater than I could have expected had I gone straight to print ... and best of all, it didn't cost anything, except a lot of time!

The mission:

My goal with this project was to create the most informative, easy-to-read, and above all, the "shortest" ophthalmology textbook ever written.

Surprisingly, there aren't that many high-yield books like this in publication. Those other (yawn) inferior textbooks are the size of Webster's Dictionary and read like the Encyclopedia Britannica. Given the dominance of these classic texts, I asked myself early on, "Is there even a need for a little eye book like mine?"

Fortunately, the positive response from my readers show that OphthoBook does fill a niche for a simple and power-packed ocular textbook that is small enough to fit in a jacket pocket.

Medical schools provide little or no ophthalmologic training in their core curriculum, and students need a concise review of ophthalmology that is approachable and fun to read. I've kept this text short for a reason – seriously, it's been hard to keep this book as brief as it is! I've been tempted many times to expand sections, add chapters, and delve into detail, but have curtailed this impulse. I've made great efforts to keep this book short and relevant for students and non-ophthalmologist. Simplicity is the book's main selling point.

The book's not perfect. It is a lighthearted overview of an extremely complicated subject, the human eye. Since this book is written primarily for medical students, many readers may find some chapters too technical and become bored. Just keep chugging through, however, and I think you'll eventually find something worthwhile, or maybe a cartoon that makes you smile.

With that "self-handicapping" out of the way, let me preface this introduction with one last qualifier for those reading the "free" version of this book: You're getting what you paid for, so "eye" hope you enjoy it!

2. Root Atlas: Online slit-lamp video atlas

www.RootAtlas.com

Root Atlas is an online collection of common eye findings, captured as high-quality videos. The eye is particularly difficult to image. Macro photography is challenging, given the reflective nature of the cornea. Video capture is even more difficult because of the light levels required for good focus.

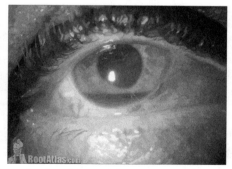

Dr. Root captured many of these videos during his residency training and helped pioneer some of the earliest stereoscopic video techniques used on the eye.

Before Root Atlas, there were few teaching videos available for students. His website is still (to our knowledge) the largest collection of slit-lamp videos out there and most of the videos are available for download for teaching purposes. These videos are used by doctors and educators worldwide in their own medical lectures. Root Atlas has even gained the attention of national media and has been used in medical television series such as The Doctors on CBS. Visit www.RootAtlas.com for more on these interesting videos.

The website draws in about 30,000 visitors every month. Some of the most popular videos include:

Corneal Foreign Body Removal - Watch Dr. Root remove a piece of metal from the eye using a needle. (1 minute)

Laser Peripheral Iridotomy - Watch as Dr. Root lasers through the iris to treat acute glaucoma. (1:15 minutes)

Asteroid Hyalosis - Want to see what floaters look like inside the eye? While harmless, these ocular "asteroids" look impressive. (48 seconds)

3. Dr. Root's Live Lecture Series

Available at OphthoBook.com and YouTube.com

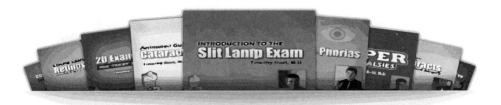

Dr. Root frequently presents his medical lectures before live audiences. Many of these lectures are available online for remote learning students.

These lectures are currently the most viewed eye presentations in the world with Dr. Root's YouTube video channel breaking 2,000,000 views.

His lectures are also available as podcasts through iTunes, with more than 100,000 lectures downloaded throughout the past year.

If you'd like to watch Dr. Root speak in front of an audience, visit OphthoBook.com or search for his videos on YouTube. Some of the most popular talks include:

Introduction to the Slit-Lamp Exam: A humorous demonstration of how the eye microscope works, and the common findings doctors look for in their patients. (24 minutes)

The Exploding Eye: An examination of traumatic eye injuries inflicted on preserved pig eyes (lasers, fireworks, chemicals) and what this can teach us about human eye injury. (29 minutes)

Cartoon Cataract Surgery: A cartoon and live video demonstration of all the steps and equipment involved in a cataract surgery. (9 minutes)

Super Eye Palsies: Video-intense explanation of nerve palsies and double vision ... complete with "super" patient examples. (30 minutes)

4. Future Root Projects

www.RootEyeNetwork.com

Dr. Root keeps himself pretty busy. He has several future publications that include:

EyeTalkRadio.com - Dr. Root is completing discussions for a talk show about the eye. This will be released globally and features basic eye topics and caller questions.

My First Cataract - An expanded version of The Cataract Handbook used in Dr. Root's practice. If you're contemplating cataract surgery ... My First Cataract is the book you need to read first!

If you'd like a notification when these projects are released, sign up for our email newsletter at:

www.RootEyeNetwork.com